# *THE DIABETES SOLUTION*

Symptoms the body feels can be determined by the human eyes.

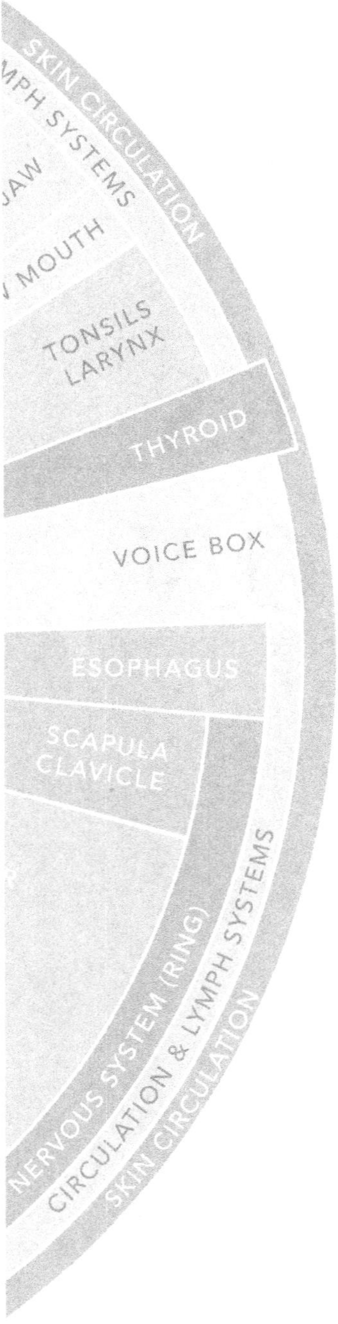

# THE DIABETES SOLUTION A 28 DAY ACTION PLAN FOR LOWERING BLOOD SUGAR NATURALLY

Ronald Delary-Simpson
&
Petrina Ten

ISBN : 9798397398978

## MEDICAL DISCLAIMER

The medical or health information in this book is provided as an information resource only, as is not to be used or relied on for any diagnostic or treatment purposes.

This information is not intended to be patient education, does not create any patient-physician relationship, and should not be used as a substitute for professional diagnosis and treatment.

The information and resources provided in this book are based on the authors' personal experiences. Any outcome, health statements or other results, are based on the authors' experiences. There is no guarantee that your experience will be the same nor will you have similar results from reading this book.

The authors reserve the right to make changes and assume no responsibility or liability whatsoever on behalf of any purchaser or reader of these materials.

## ACKNOWLEDGEMENTS

Thank you to our family, friends, team members and customers who have believed in us and supported us throughout the years.

Many thanks to all our mentors, past and present, who have encouraged and taught us so much on how to serve better.

We are grateful to everyone who took part in our surveys and/or gave us feedback and assistance during the writing and publishing of this book.

To all our readers who have spent their time reading, learning and implementing from this book, we appreciate you.

We look forward to connecting with each one of you soon.

Many beautiful things cannot be seen or touched;
they are felt with the heart.

What you have done for us is one of them and we
thank you from the bottom of our hearts.

# PRAISE

Ronald and Petrina are a powerful couple with a gift for helping people achieve, what conventional mainstream medicine would term “the impossible”. More importantly, they have a catalogue of results to prove it – and that’s how I like to judge, by results.

One must experience the paradigm-shifting health and wellness knowledge that Ronald and Petrina possess for themselves because it is, indeed, an experience that has the potential to change a daunting set of failing health circumstances to one of hope. The fact that my brother is still alive today and now thriving in excellent health is proof of that.

Ronald and Petrina will educate and provide a clear, proven path for you to follow to achieve a powerful transformation from whatever ails you to complete health and wellness. It’s a level of service that, in my experience, you just won’t get from any of today’s GPs. I cannot say enough good about them. Highly recommended.

*Darren-Lee Joseph (Jamaica)*

My husband and I were in Ibiza for a short holiday where we met Petrina. On one of the days, we were having nausea and headache. Petrina's knowledge on natural remedies is amazing. We took her recommendations and felt a lot better after several minutes. She is wonderful in providing these tips and care!

*Yaling Zhang (China & Netherlands)*

My nutrition has improved greatly! The Iridology examination was an eye opener (pun intended) to the possibilities of a sustainable healthy lifestyle.

*Dr Folake Oluokun (USA)*

A calm, cool, healing environment. It is one of those very rare places where you feel better before even arriving. To me, that is the essence of true healers. They combine advice on nutrition, gardening, and cooking for each person. That's the whole food chain. Ronald and Petrina love to share their immense knowledge with like-minded people wanting to change and transform their lives.

*John Burger (United Kingdom)*

I am so grateful for the heartfelt care, love, genuine energy and outstanding knowledge and healing service that Petrina and Ronald at Planet Wellness gave me. Their depth and breadth of knowledge, experience and wisdom in nutrition and iridology is outstanding.

I felt so listened to, cared for, helped. They shared amazing information and pointers on long-term disease prevention and wellbeing-knowledge based on their years of research, education, experience, and real love to help others.

Their kindness and generosity in what they give, how they care and time they spend truly touched me. I have learned so much from this healing couple about nutrition and blown away about Iridology in diagnosing and managing conditions.

Thank you, Petrina, and Ronald, for your passion, service, mission and for helping so many live healthier and empowered lives. I would absolutely recommend their service. Many blessings and best wishes to you both.

*Dr Thuvaraka Vetpillai (Sri Lanka)*

The two weeks of detoxification has done wonders to my body. Thank you so much for your meal tips.

*Pawel C (Poland)*

My family and I are extremely pleased and grateful for all the support we have received and are still receiving from our Iridology appointments. It takes a lot of willpower to change one's lifestyle. We had a lot to adjust to.

What made it much easier is that Ronald and Petrina included the children and helped them realise through their own eye images and kinesiology, how much is going on within us. Now it's a family affair.
I am so grateful as we have tried to improve our meals before but was never consistent. With all the resources we now have access to and ability to ask questions is wonderful for all of us. We have also made gradual changes to brown rice, organic celery, and spelt flour.

Thank you for revolutionising the way we see food, which is our medicine.

*Sekinat Yakub (Nigeria)*

Petrina and Ronald analysed the eye photos of my family remotely. They were able to identify root causes of our illnesses and organ weaknesses.

This has saved us a lot of time. Their detailed knowledge of nutrition is helping us be healthier. Their after care and customer support is also amazing. Highly recommend you reach out and have a chat with them.

*Sanae Ben Hammou (Morocco & Turkey)*

I would highly recommend Planet Wellness. Ronald's knowledge and years of experience with Iridology and Nutrition is incredible. He is a master in this healing modality.

If you want to make improvements to your health, get in touch for holistic guidance in transforming your health and wellbeing.

*Belinda Wood (Australia)*

My whole family has had the benefit of Iridology and Nutrition sessions with Ronald and Petrina. As a clinician of 32 years, this was the best consultation I have ever had.

Our health care system fails to address the core of our illnesses and for many, what we eat is making us sick. We have embraced the nutritional recommendations and are seeing improvements.

Having had Iridology before as a taster session, this was detailed and the findings in sync with my health issues. I highly recommend everyone to have a session as it will leave a permanent imprint for change which is not only physical and practical but psychological.

*Arlene C (Venezeula & Trinidad)*

Ronald and Petrina are kind and approachable with all clarifications. They identify the root cause of the underlying health problems and suggest the exact nutrition to intake. I recommend them as the go to people for any underlying health issues.

*Nishanth Ramanathan (India)*

We have known Ronald and Petrina since 2017. We often wonder what our family's health and nutrition would be like if Sam had not seen "gardener Ronald" on that fateful day in June.

All the praises in this book are 100% true and deserved. The value of knowledge and insight we have obtained from them on all things relating to the state of body and mind (and many more) are unparalleled.

Friends and family who have also had the opportunity to attend an Iridology session or seek out health and nutrition advice have never been disappointed either.

If you value your health, make time to get in touch or at least implement the gems they have shared in this book and on their social media for Wellness related tips.

We are privileged to have access to personal nutritionists who have taught us how to prevent and manage disease with nutrition. Cheers to letting thy food be thy medicine.

Michelle and Sam Mensah
(Kenya and Ghana)

# PREFACE

## WHAT INSPIRED THIS BOOK?

We specialise in avoiding and reversing Diabetes Type 2 naturally. Many of our customers have been impressed by our vast knowledge, and more importantly results achieved from following our recommendations. We have been asked to document our knowledge so that we can reach a wider audience and help more people who are ready to be helped. It will also serve as our legacy to future generations.

## WHAT TOOK US SO LONG?

As you can imagine, life often gets in the way and various other matters take priority. There is also the fear of being judged or criticised by those who may not agree with our proven knowledge or recommendations.

Before we realise, another day, week, month, and year has passed us by. We are very grateful to our main mentor, Mr James Nicholson for encouraging us to write and publish this book in under 8 weeks.

It is a great achievement as apart from writing and publishing this book, we also managed to carry on with our daily lives, including running a Wellness practice, attending events and travels that were already pre-booked months in advance.

You may not agree with everything that is shared in this book and there may even be typos or grammatical errors. We appreciate if you could reach out to us via

hello@planetwellness.co.uk

if you pick up any mistakes or need further clarifications.

## ABOUT THIS BOOK

This book has been written with the reader in mind. Based on years of experience of helping many Diabetic and Pre-Diabetic patients, we have done our best to explain our content in layperson's terms. We have shared information you are unlikely to receive from your own Doctor or Nurse. The Medical Professionals are bound by tight time and cost budgets. They normally only have 10 minutes allocated per patient per appointment.

## WHO IS THIS BOOK FOR?

Whether you are Diabetic, Pre-Diabetic or not, this book is a recommended read. Why? Not because we have written it. It is because the information we share will help you remain healthy if you are. If you are already Diabetic or Pre-Diabetic, then following our recommendations will help you lower your blood sugar naturally within days.

If you are taking any chemical medication to control or lower your blood sugar, then you may over time also be able to wean off these. Please do consult your medical practitioner before weaning yourself off any chemical medication prescribed by them.

*Take care of your body. It's the only place you have to live.*

*Jim Rohn – American entrepreneur*

## ABOUT THE AUTHORS

Ronald Delary-Simpson and Petrina Ten live in London, United Kingdom. They run a Wellness Clinic called Planet Wellness. They have been successfully helping customers worldwide for many years. They have also been regular guests on TV and radio stations for many years.

Some customers even travel from overseas to visit them for their non-invasive Wellness Iridology and Smart Nutrition consultation services. Their clinic is well appreciated for its very calm space and organic garden.

Ronald and Petrina are very much focused on achieving results vs time and money focused. They will do their best to help you achieve and maintain your Wellness goals. No disease or illness is too challenging. If you do not give up on your health and keep following their recommendations, they too will not give up on guiding you towards the best pathway of healing.

They currently have two YouTube channels:

www.youtube.com/@planetwellness

www.youtube.com/@planetwellnessiridology

where they publish new videos several times a week on Wellness related topics.
Do also check out their website where they publish new blogs every week.

www.planetwellness.co.uk

## HOW TO GET THE BEST RESULTS FROM THIS BOOK?

This book consists of a 28 Day Action Plan (or 28 main chapters) for lowering blood sugar naturally. We do understand you may be busy and may not be able to read a chapter each consecutive day or implement what you have read and learnt immediately.

Do attempt to read at least a chapter daily. Depending on your reading speed and skills, set aside say 20 minutes just as you would set aside time to work, commute or relax.

This is YOUR HEALTH, and it is important that you give it priority.

We recommend you read this book and each chapter more than once, in fact at least 3 times to digest, understand and implement its contents properly.
We have left a notes section at the end of each chapter. If you wish, write down any points, action plan or reminders. Studies have proven that writing by hand forces your brain to process information in a more detailed way. You are therefore more likely to remember things and get things done. Do also complete the recommended exercises at the end of some of the chapters.

# TABLE OF CONTENTS

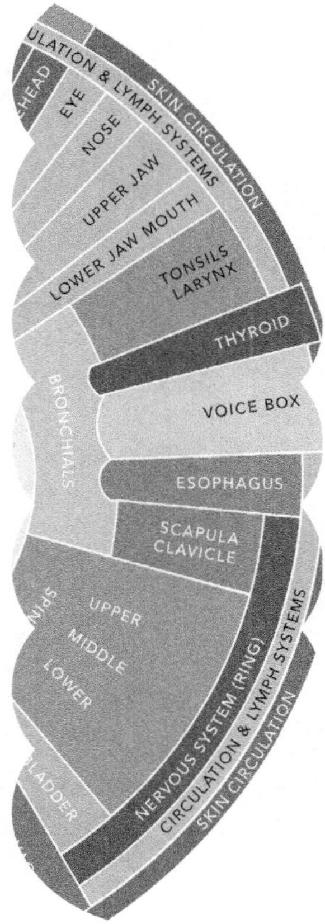

# TABLE OF CONTENTS

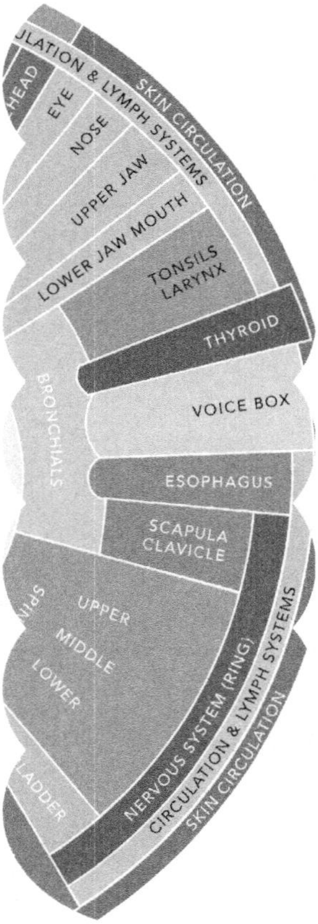

# TABLE OF CONTENTS

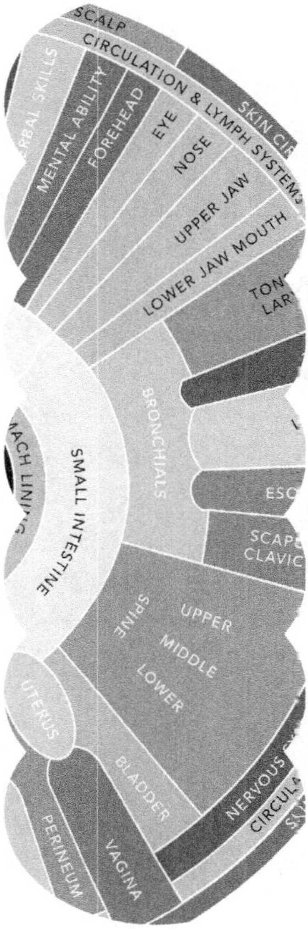

# TABLE OF CONTENTS

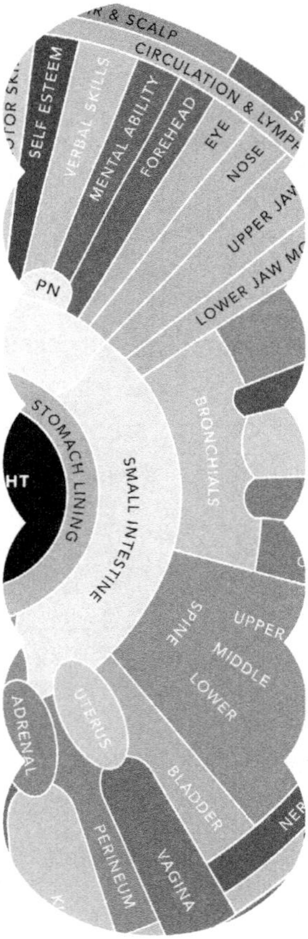

# TABLE OF CONTENTS

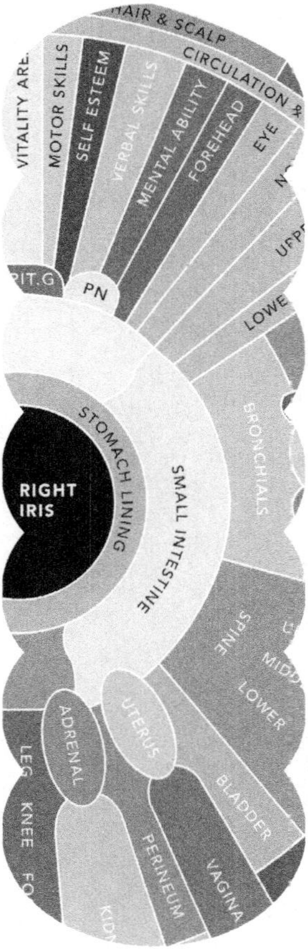

# *Introduction*

# *INTRODUCTION*

## UNDERSTANDING DIABETES AND ITS IMPACT ON HEALTH

In this chapter, we will delve into the fundamentals of diabetes, exploring its different types, the location, and roles of the pancreas, as well as the global prevalence of this chronic condition. Additionally, we will shed light on the long-term dangers that can arise from untreated diabetes, such as amputations and impaired wound healing.

## TYPES OF DIABETES

Diabetes is a metabolic disorder characterized by elevated blood sugar levels. There are primarily three types of diabetes: type 1 diabetes, type 2 diabetes, and gestational diabetes.

## TYPE 1 DIABETES

Type 1 diabetes is an autoimmune condition where the immune system mistakenly attacks the insulin-producing cells in the pancreas.

As a result, the pancreas produces little to no insulin. Insulin is a hormone that allows glucose to enter cells for energy production. Individuals with type 1 diabetes require insulin therapy for survival.

## TYPE 2 DIABETES

Type 2 diabetes is the most common form of diabetes, accounting for most cases worldwide. It occurs when the body becomes resistant to insulin or fails to produce enough insulin to maintain normal blood sugar levels.

Lifestyle factors such as obesity, sedentary behaviour, and poor dietary habits contribute significantly to the development of type 2 diabetes.

## GESTATIONAL DIABETES

Gestational diabetes occurs during pregnancy when hormonal changes impair insulin action. Although it typically resolves after childbirth, women who have had gestational diabetes are at a higher risk of developing type 2 diabetes later in life.

## THE PANCREAS AND ITS ROLES

When we meet patients who have been diagnosed as Pre-Diabetic or Diabetic, there is one main thing that concerns us the most. Very rarely does the Doctor or Nurse explain to their patients where the pancreas is, what it looks like and its role.

The pancreas, a glandular organ located in the abdomen, plays a vital role in maintaining blood sugar levels through the production of insulin and other digestive enzymes.

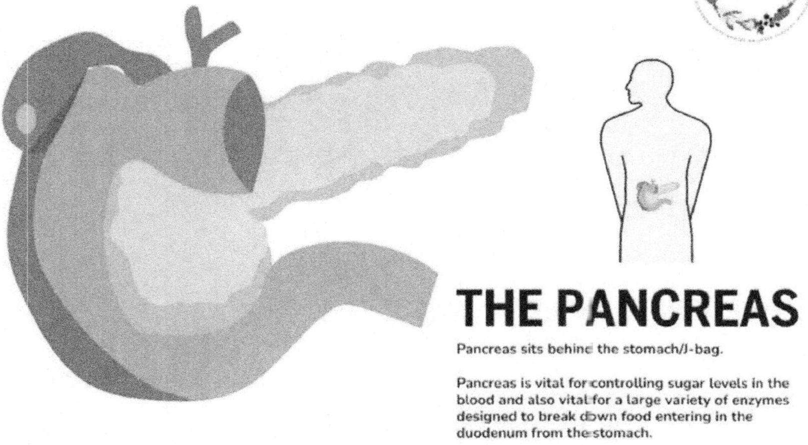


In our free guide Best Ways To Treat Diabetes, we also explain the importance of strengthening at least 4 other key organs, apart from the Pancreas to prevent or treat Diabetes.

**INSULIN PRODUCTION**

Within the pancreas, specialized cells called beta cells are responsible for producing and secreting insulin into the bloodstream. Insulin enables cells to absorb glucose from the bloodstream, thereby reducing blood sugar levels.

## DIGESTIVE ENZYMES

The pancreas also produces digestive enzymes that aid in the breakdown and absorption of nutrients from food, including proteins, fats, and carbohydrates.

## GLOBAL PREVALENCE OF DIABETES

Diabetes is a global health concern, affecting millions of people worldwide. According to the International Diabetes Federation, approximately 463 million adults (20-79 years) were living with diabetes in 2019, accounting for around 9.3% of the global population. It is estimated to rise to 10.2% (578 million) by 2030 and 10.9% (700 million) by 2045. The prevalence is higher in urban (10.8%) than rural (7.2%) areas, an in higher income (10.4%) than lower income countries (4%).

Alarmingly, it is estimated that about half of these individuals remain undiagnosed, unknowingly living with uncontrolled blood sugar levels.

Diabetes is increasing so steadily that every third person will be suffering from it soon. If we would only realise that we have our life and health in our own hands, and if we could know where to seek our health, it would be the most wonderful thing in the world.

## LONG-TERM DANGERS OF UNTREATED DIABETES

When diabetes is left untreated or poorly managed, it can lead to severe complications, including:

### AMPUTATIONS

High blood sugar levels can damage blood vessels and nerves, particularly in the extremities. Over time, this can result in poor circulation, nerve damage, and non-healing foot ulcers, increasing the risk of lower limb amputations.

### IMPAIRED WOUND HEALING

Diabetes can impair the body's natural healing process, making it difficult for wounds to heal. Even minor cuts or blisters can become serious infections if not promptly and properly treated.

### EYESIGHT AND OTHER COMPLICATIONS

Untreated diabetes can have a profound impact on eyesight and overall health. Prolonged high blood sugar levels can damage the blood vessels in the retina, leading to a condition called diabetic retinopathy. This progressive eye disease can cause vision impairment and, if left untreated, may even result in blindness.

Diabetes can also increase the risk of developing other eye problems, such as cataracts and glaucoma. Furthermore, uncontrolled diabetes can affect the health of the kidneys, leading to diabetic nephropathy, a condition that impairs kidney function and may ultimately require dialysis or kidney transplantation.

Additionally, diabetes increases the risk of cardiovascular diseases, such as heart attacks and strokes, due to the detrimental effects of high blood sugar levels on blood vessels and the heart. Unmanaged diabetes can also lead to nerve damage (neuropathy), affecting various parts of the body, including the feet and hands, resulting in numbness, pain, and potential complications like foot ulcers and infections.

Overall, these long-term complications highlight the critical importance of effective diabetes management to safeguard not only eyesight but also the overall well-being and quality of life of individuals living with diabetes.

## SUMMARY

Understanding the various types of diabetes, the role of the pancreas, and the potential consequence of untreated diabetes is crucial in comprehending the importance of managing this condition effectively. By equipping ourselves with knowledge, we can take proactive steps toward improving our health and achieving optimal blood sugar control.

**NOTES :**

.................................................................................................

.................................................................................................

.................................................................................................

.................................................................................................

.................................................................................................

.................................................................................................

.................................................................................................

.................................................................................................

.................................................................................................

.................................................................................................

.................................................................................................

.................................................................................................

.................................................................................................

.................................................................................................

.................................................................................................

.................................................................................................

.................................................................................................

.................................................................................................

.................................................................................................

.................................................................................................

.................................................................................................

.................................................................................................

.................................................................................................

# *Chapter 1*

## *The Power of Mindset and Shifting Your Perspective on Diabetes*

*Welcome to the exciting journey of exploring the power of mindset and how it can transform your perspective on diabetes.*

*In this chapter, we'll dive into some amazing insights that will not only make you smile but also empower you to take control of your health.*

*So, fasten your seatbelts and get ready for a fun and easy ride!*

*Chapter 1*

## THE FAMILY LEGACY MYTH

First things first, let's debunk a common misconception. Having a family history of diabetes doesn't mean you're destined to follow in their footsteps. Yes, genetics can play a role, but they're not the be-all and end-all.

Research has shown that lifestyle choices, such as exercise and healthier eating, can significantly reduce the risk of developing diabetes, even if it runs in the family. So, wave goodbye to the "inevitability" mindset and get ready to embrace the power you hold to make a positive difference.

**HUMAN BEING COMPOSITE**

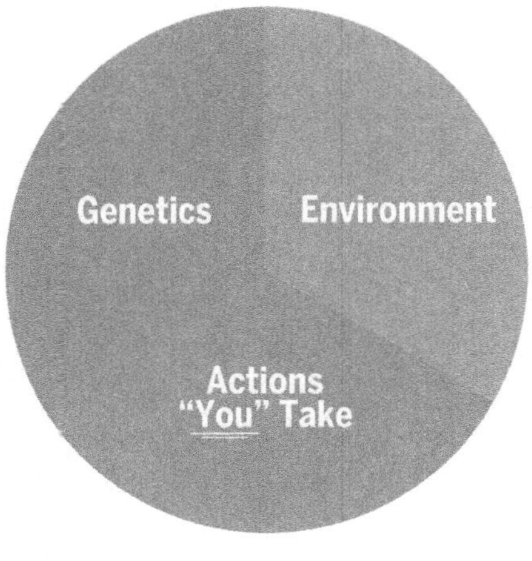

## EMPOWERING CHOICES

Here's the thing; your mindset is like a superhero cape that you can wear every day. It's about believing that you have the power to make choices that support your health and well-being.

So, instead of dwelling on what you can't do, focus on what you can do. Celebrate the small victories, whether it's choosing a nutritious snack or going for a walk.

These seemingly tiny actions can have a tremendous impact on your journey towards preventing or managing diabetes.

## THE THREE CS: CURIOSITY, COMMITMENT, AND CONSISTENCY:

To unlock the power of mindset, let's introduce the three Cs:

Curiosity is the spark that ignites the desire to learn and understand more about diabetes and how it affects your body. It's about asking questions, seeking knowledge, and staying open to new possibilities.

Commitment means making a heartfelt decision to prioritise your health and well-being. It's about making conscious choices that align with your goals and values.

Consistency is the secret sauce that brings it all together. Small, consistent actions add up to significant long-term results. Remember, it's not about being perfect; it's about being persistent and making progress.

*Small disciplines repeated with consistency daily lead to great achievements gained slowly over time.*

*John Maxwell*

## EMBRACE THE ADVENTURE

Managing diabetes doesn't have to be a chore. It can be an exciting adventure filled with new discoveries, delicious food, and delightful activ ties. Explore different types of exercises and find the ones that bring you joy.

Experiment with wholesome, flavourful recipes (some of our recommended recipes are in Chapter 8) that nourish your body and tantalize your taste buds. Surround yourself with a support network of friends, family, or fellow diabetes warriors who can share experiences, provide encouragement, and celebrate your successes.

Embrace the journey with a playful and positive mindset, and you'll discover that managing diabetes can be an opportunity for persona growth and empowerment.

## SUMMARY

Congratulations!

You've completed reading the first chapter of this incredible journey, where we've explored the power of mindset and shattered the myth that diabetes is an inevitable family legacy.

Remember, YOU hold the key to making choices that support your health and well-being. Curiosity, commitment, and consistency will be your steadfast companions as you navigate the adventure of preventing or managing diabetes.

So, put on your superhero cape of mindset, embrace the power within you, and get ready to unlock a world of possibilities!

## RECOMMENDED EXERCISES :

1.WRITE DOWN AT LEAST ONE HEALTHIER CHOICE YOU ARE GOING TO IMPLEMENT TODAY.

FOR EXAMPLE, WALK A BIT MORE BY TAKING THE STAIRS INSTEAD OF THE LIFT OR ESCALATOR OR WALK INSTEAD OF DRIVING.

..............................................................................................
..............................................................................................
..............................................................................................
..............................................................................................
..............................................................................................
..............................................................................................
..............................................................................................
..............................................................................................
..............................................................................................
..............................................................................................
..............................................................................................
..............................................................................................
..............................................................................................
..............................................................................................
..............................................................................................
..............................................................................................

2. WRITE DOWN A HURDLE YOU MAY HAVE TO OVERCOME WITH REGARDS TO YOUR HEALTHIER CHOICE.

FOR EXAMPLE, UPSETTING SOMEONE BY NOT HAVING THAT UNHEALTHY DESSERT.

..........................................................................................

..........................................................................................

..........................................................................................

..........................................................................................

..........................................................................................

..........................................................................................

..........................................................................................

..........................................................................................

..........................................................................................

..........................................................................................

..........................................................................................

..........................................................................................

..........................................................................................

..........................................................................................

..........................................................................................

..........................................................................................

3. WRITE DOWN HOW YOU INTEND TO OVERCOME THIS HURDLE SO YOU ARE READY WHEN FACED WITH IT.
FOR EXAMPLE, EXPLAIN TO THE PERSON THAT YOUR HEALTH IS IMPORTANT AND YOU WOULD APPRECIATE THAT THEY SUPPORT YOU ON YOUR JOURNEY TO IMPROVED WELLNESS.

........................................................................................................
........................................................................................................
........................................................................................................
........................................................................................................
........................................................................................................
........................................................................................................
........................................................................................................
........................................................................................................
........................................................................................................
........................................................................................................
........................................................................................................
........................................................................................................
........................................................................................................
........................................................................................................
........................................................................................................
........................................................................................................

*Every accomplishment starts with the decision to try.*
*Brian Littrell*

*Singer-Music Artist*

**NOTES :**

**NOTES :**

# *Chapter 2*

## *Setting Clear Goals for Blood Sugar Control*

*Well done on embarking on this exciting journey towards blood sugar control!*

*In this chapter, we'll dive into the importance of setting clear goals and how they can empower you to overcome cultural influences, peer pressure, unhealthy advertisements, and the pressure to eat on the go.*

*Get ready to define your path towards success!*

## Chapter 2

### UNRAVELLING CULTURAL AND TRADITIONAL INFLUENCES

Cultural and traditional upbringing often play a significant role in our eating habits. However, it's essential to recognise that not all cultural practices align with optimal blood sugar control.

Challenge any misconceptions and myths surrounding certain foods and their impact on your health.

Educate yourself about healthy alternatives and traditional dishes that can be modified to fit your needs. We share some of our personal recipes in Chapter 8.

Remember, you have the power to redefine your relationship with food and create a healthier cultural fusion that supports your blood sugar goals.

“

*Goals help you channel your energy into action.*

*Les Brown*
*Motivational Speaker*

”

## NAVIGATING PEER PRESSURE

Peer pressure can be challenging, especially when it comes to food choices. Whether it's social gatherings or outings with friends, the temptation to indulge in less healthy options may arise.

The key is to stand firm in your commitment to blood sugar control while finding ways to navigate these situations. Communicate your goals with friends and loved ones, explaining the importance of their support.

Seek out like-minded individuals who share your health values and can provide encouragement when faced with peer pressure.

Remember, prioritising your well-being is not only a personal choice but also an inspiration for those around you.

*Chapter 2*

## TAMING THE TEMPTATIONS OF UNHEALTHY ADVERTISEMENTS

Unhealthy food advertisements bombard us daily, enticing us with tempting treats that can wreak havoc on blood sugar levels. Being aware of their influence is the first step towards overcoming their impact.

Practice mindful consumption of media, recognizing the persuasive nature of advertisements. Limit exposure to such ads by seeking out educational content, positive role models, and healthy lifestyle influencers who promote balanced eating habits.

Surround yourself with visuals and messages that reinforce your commitment to blood sugar control, making it easier to resist the seduction of unhealthy choices.

## OVERCOMING THE PRESSURE TO EAT ON THE GO

In today's fast-paced world, eating on the go has become the norm for many. This often leads to impulsive and unhealthy food choices that can sabotage blood sugar control.

Release yourself from this cycle by planning and prioritising meal preparation in advance. Set aside dedicated time for meal planning, grocery shopping, and cooking nutritious meals in advance.

Have nutritious snacks and drinks such as fruit, nuts, seeds, mineral water, coconut water or herbal teas with you when commuting. This will stop you from buying unhealthy food on the go and even save you a lot of money in the longer term as eating out adds to your food bills.

By having healthy options readily available, you can resist the pressure to grab quick but detrimental alternatives. Remember, nourishing your body with balanced meals is a valuable investment in your long-term health and blood sugar management.

## SUMMARY

As you conclude this chapter, you now understand the significance of setting clear goals for blood sugar control. By releasing yourself from incorrect cultural influences, overcoming peer pressure, taming the temptations of unhealthy advertisements, and resisting the pressure to eat on the go, you are empowering yourself to achieve optimal blood sugar management.

Remember, your goals are unique to you, and with commitment and perseverance, you have the power to redefine your relationship with food and embrace a lifestyle that supports your well-being.

So, define your path, set those goals, and get ready to embark on an incredible journey towards blood sugar control!

## RECOMMENDED EXERCISES :

1.WRITE DOWN AT LEAST ONE HEALTHIER FOOD CHOICE YOU ARE GOING TO IMPLEMENT TODAY.
FOR EXAMPLE, SWAPPING EATING CRISPS WITH EATING A RED APPLE INSTEAD.

..............................................................................

..............................................................................

..............................................................................

..............................................................................

..............................................................................

..............................................................................

..............................................................................

..............................................................................

..............................................................................

..............................................................................

..............................................................................

..............................................................................

..............................................................................

..............................................................................

..............................................................................

..............................................................................

2 WRITE DOWN AT LEAST CULTURAL FOOD THAT YOU NOW KNOW IS UNHEALTHY AND THE IMPROVISATION YOU ARE GOING TO IMPLEMENT GOING FORWARD.

FOR EXAMPLE, EATING HEALTHIER AND MORE NUTRITIOUS BROWN RICE INSTEAD OF WHITE RICE.

..........................................................................

..........................................................................

..........................................................................

..........................................................................

..........................................................................

..........................................................................

..........................................................................

..........................................................................

..........................................................................

..........................................................................

..........................................................................

..........................................................................

..........................................................................

..........................................................................

..........................................................................

..........................................................................

3 .WRITE DOWN AT LEAST ONE HEALTHIER FOOD OR DRINK THAT YOU ARE GOING TO STOCK UP ON GOING FORWARD. FOR EXAMPLE, GREEN OR HERBAL TEA INSTEAD OF BLACK TEA. BROWN SUGAR OR RAW HONEY INSTEAD OF WHITE SUGAR.

*Success is the product of daily habits.*

*James Clear*
*Author*

**NOTES :**

**NOTES :**

# *Chapter 3*

# *Creating a Positive Diabetes Action Plan*

*This is the chapter that will ignite your motivation and empower you to create a positive diabetes action plan!*

*In this easy-to-read and fun-filled chapter, we'll explore how you can overcome the challenges of busyness and discipline while crafting a feasible and exciting action plan.*

*Get ready to unleash your inner superhero and take charge of your diabetes management!*

## EMBRACING FEASIBILITY

Creating an action plan may seem daunting, especially if you're juggling a busy schedule or struggling with discipline. Relax, because feasibility is the name of the game!

Remember that your action plan should align with your lifestyle, making it easier to integrate into your daily routine. Start small, focusing on achievable steps that you can consistently incorporate into your life.

It's better to take baby steps than to overwhelm yourself with drastic changes. By embracing feasibility, you set yourself up for success!

YOU CAN DO THIS!

*"If you believe in it,*
*and you believe in it*
*hard,*
*it is impossible to fail.*

*Ray Kroc*
*American*
*Businessman"*

## TIME-SAVING STRATEGIES

For those caught in the whirlwind of a busy lifestyle, finding time for diabetes management can be a challenge. However, with a little creativity and planning, it's doable!

Look for time-saving strategies such as meal prepping on weekends, utilizing slow cookers or easy recipes for quick and healthy meals. Set aside dedicated time for physical activity. By making efficient use of your time, you can prioritise your health without sacrificing other important aspects of your life.

## THE POWER OF ACCOUNTABILITY

Sometimes, discipline can waver, and that's okay. You're only human! But here's the secret: accountability can be a game-changer. Seek support from family, friends, or even online communities dedicated to diabetes management. Share your action plan with someone you trust and ask them to hold you accountable.

Consider joining exercise classes or finding a workout buddy who can keep you motivated. Remember, you don't have to go at it alone.

Together, we're stronger!

**TEAM**
Together
Everyone
Achieves
More

Celebrate Progress, Not Perfection:

One of the keys to maintaining a positive mindset is celebrating your progress, no matter how small. Rather than striving for perfection, focus on consistently moving forward. Each healthy choice you make, every blood sugar reading within range, and every step towards a more balanced lifestyle is a victory worth celebrating. Embrace the journey with self-compassion and acknowledge that setbacks are a natural part of the process. Be kind to yourself and use setbacks as opportunities to learn and grow.

## SUMMARY

Congratulations on reaching the end of this fun and inspiring chapter! You now know that creating a positive diabetes action plan is feasible, even for the busiest of individuals or those lacking discipline.

By embracing feasibility, implementing time-saving strategies, harnessing the power of accountability, and celebrating progress, you're well on your way to successfully managing your diabetes naturally.

Remember, you are capable of incredible things, and with determination and the support of those around you, your action plan will become a vibrant roadmap towards a healthier and happier life.

So, put on your superhero cape, embrace the possibilities, and create your positive diabetes action plan today!

*"What you do every day matters more than what you do once in a while.*

*Gretchen Rubin*
*American Author"*

## RECOMMENDED EXERCISES

1. WRITE DOWN AT LEAST ONE ACTION PLAN YOU ARE GOING TO IMPLEMENT TODAY.

FOR EXAMPLE, BRINGING A HEALTHIER PACKED LUNCH TO WORK INSTEAD OF BUYING A TAKEAWAY OR EATING OUT.

...............................................................................

...............................................................................

...............................................................................

...............................................................................

...............................................................................

...............................................................................

...............................................................................

...............................................................................

...............................................................................

...............................................................................

...............................................................................

...............................................................................

...............................................................................

...............................................................................

...............................................................................

2. WRITE DOWN THE NAME OF AT LEAST ONE PERSON WHO CAN HELP HOLD YOU ACCOUNTABLE FOR THESE LIFESTYE CHANGES AND HOW THIS WILL BE ACHIEVED.

FOR EXAMPLE, A WORK COLLEAGUE OR FAMILY MEMBER BY SENDING REMINDERS OR KEEPING EACH OTHER UPDATED ON THE LIFESTYLE CHANGES.

..............................................................................
..............................................................................
..............................................................................
..............................................................................
..............................................................................
..............................................................................
..............................................................................
..............................................................................
..............................................................................
..............................................................................
..............................................................................
..............................................................................
..............................................................................
..............................................................................
..............................................................................

3. WRITE DOWN HOW YOU WILL REWARD YOURSELF FOR EACH ACHIEVEMENT.

IT COULD BE AS SIMPLE AS THE OLD SCHOOL "PLACE A GOLD STAR OR TICK" ON YOUR ACHIEVEMENT MONITOR BOARD OR TREATING YOURSELF TO A NEW OUTFIT.

......................................................................................................

......................................................................................................

......................................................................................................

......................................................................................................

......................................................................................................

......................................................................................................

......................................................................................................

......................................................................................................

......................................................................................................

......................................................................................................

......................................................................................................

......................................................................................................

......................................................................................................

......................................................................................................

......................................................................................................

......................................................................................................

“

*Today is your opportunity to build the tomorrow you want.*

*Ken Poirot*
Author

”

## NOTES :

**NOTES :**

# *Chapter 4*

## *NON-INVASIVE HEALTH CHECKS*

*Welcome to the fascinating world of non-invasive health checks, where we explore the intriguing practice of iridology!*

*In this fun and easy-to-read chapter, we'll dive into what iridology is all about, how it can help detect health concerns like diabetes before symptoms arise, and its role in identifying weaknesses in other key organs.*

*Get ready to open your eyes to a new way of understanding your health!*

*Chapter 4*

## THE EYES: WINDOWS TO OUR HEALTH

You may have heard the saying that the eyes are the windows to the soul. Well, they're also the windows to our health! In the past, doctors used to pay close attention to our eyes during examinations, recognizing that changes in the eyes can reveal valuable information about our overall well-being. However, due to time constraints in modern medical practices, this aspect of eye examination has taken a back seat. Relax, because that's where iridology comes into the picture.

## EXPLORING IRIDOLOGY

So, what exactly is iridology? It's a non-invasive health assessment technique that involves studying the iris, the coloured part of the eye, to gain insights into a person's health. Iridologists believe that different areas of the iris correspond to specific organs and body systems. By examining the patterns, colours, and markings in the iris, iridologists can identify potential health concerns and weaknesses in the body.

## EARLY DETECTION OF DIABETES

One of the fascinating aspects of iridology is its potential to detect health issues like diabetes before symptoms manifest. By examining specific signs in the iris, such as discolorations or markings, iridologists can provide early warnings that may prompt further diagnostic testing. This early detection can be instrumental in initiating proactive measures and lifestyle changes to prevent or manage diabetes effectively.

## A HOLISTIC PERSPECTIVE

Iridology is not limited to detecting potential issues with the pancreas, the organ associated with diabetes. It takes a holistic approach by examining the entire iris to identify weaknesses in other key organs and systems.

For instance, an iridologist may detect signs of liver weakness, which can be crucial as liver health plays a significant role in blood sugar regulation.

By addressing weaknesses in various organs, you can potentially prevent conditions like diabetes from developing in the first place.

## THE FUN SIDE OF IRIDOLOGY

Now, let's add a touch of fun to the mix! Think of iridology as a playful detective game where you get to explore the intricate patterns and colours in your eyes.

It's like unlocking hidden messages about your health. Embrace this exciting adventure, as understanding your body's unique iris markings can empower you to make informed decisions and take proactive steps towards your well-being.

Remember, iridology is just one tool in your health toolkit, complementing conventional medical practices and providing additional insights.

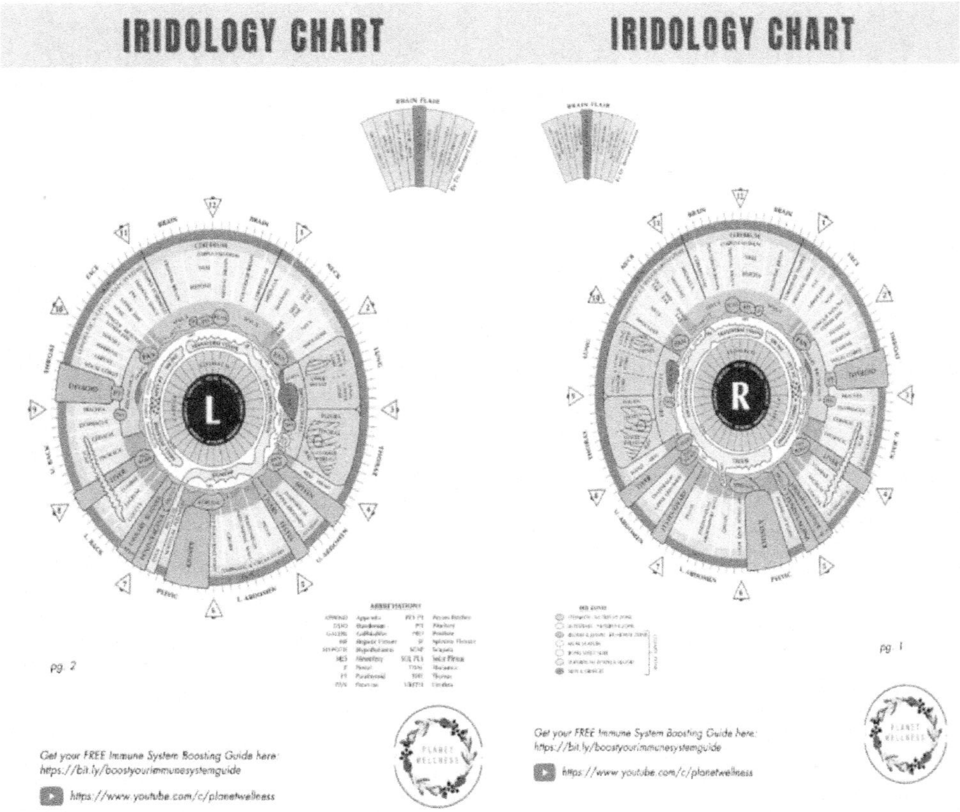


With Iridology, your eyes are the window to your body!

If you curious to know more about Iridology and how it may help you, reach out and book a free 15-minute discovery call with us via:

https://calendly.com/wellnessiridology

## SUMMARY

Well done on delving into the world of iridology! You now understand that iridology is a non-invasive health check that can provide valuable insights into your well-being.

It has the potential to detect health concerns like diabetes before symptoms arise and identify weaknesses in key organs beyond the pancreas. Remember, iridology is a holistic approach to understanding your health, and while it adds a fun twist to your wellness journey, it should be used in conjunction with conventional medical advice.

So, open your eyes wide and embrace the colourful and intricate world of iridology—it might just reveal fascinating aspects of your health that you never knew existed!

**NOTES :**

# *Chapter 5*

## *The Role of Nutrition in Controlling Blood Sugar Levels*

*Welcome to the chapter that will make healthy eating a fun and delicious adventure!*

*In this easy-to-read and captivating chapter, we'll explore the vital role of nutrition in controlling blood sugar levels. Get ready to discover how the right foods, drinks, and supplements can be your superpower in managing diabetes while avoiding the dangers of chemical medication.*

*So, let's dig in and savour the journey to optimal nutrition!*

## NOURISHING YOUR BODY WITH REAL FOOD

Nutrition plays a pivotal role in managing blood sugar levels. The foundation of a healthy meal lies in consuming real, whole foods. Fill your plate with fresh fruits, vegetables, lean proteins, whole grains, and healthy fats. These foods provide essential nutrients, fibre, and antioxidants that promote stable blood sugar levels, better insulin sensitivity, and overall well-being.

## QUENCHING YOUR THIRST MINDFULLY

Drinks can have a significant impact on blood sugar levels, so it's important to be mindful of what you sip. Choose mineral water, herbal teas, and sugar-free beverages to stay hydrated. Beware of sugary drinks like sodas and fruit juices with added sugar, which can cause spikes in blood sugar.

If you crave a hint of sweetness, infuse your water with fresh fruits or herbs for a delightful and healthy twist.

## SUPPLEMENTING WISELY

Supplements can complement a well-balanced meal. However, you need to remember that these are called supplements for this main reason. It is to "supplement" your lifestyle and healthier meal intake. Supplements are not magic fix me pills to be taken to fix your poor food choices.

Keep in mind that supplements should never replace nutritious whole foods but rather serve as an additional support system when needed.

Do also remember that supplements, even the very well-known and advertised brands may not always be the best quality. Most of us make our purchase decisions based on price.

Remember that you often need to pay a bit more for quality and when it comes to our health, we only have one body.

## DITCHING THE CHEMICAL MEDICATION TRAP

While medication can be necessary for some individuals, it's important to be aware of the potential dangers of relying solely on chemical medication to manage blood sugar.

Over-reliance on medications can mask the root causes of high blood sugar levels without addressing the underlying meal and lifestyle factors. By prioritising nutrition, you can potentially reduce or even eliminate the need for excessive medication, leading to improved overall health.

## MAKING HEALTHY EATING IRRESISTIBLE

Now, let's add some fun and excitement to healthy eating! Explore the world of flavours, textures, and colours by experimenting with wholesome ingredients. Spice up your meals with herbs and spices, try new recipes that feature nutritious and delicious ingredients, and involve friends and family in cooking adventures.

By making healthy eating enjoyable and social, you'll naturally gravitate towards nourishing options.

## OUTSMARTING THE JUNK AND PROCESSED FOODS

Junk and highly processed foods may be tempting, but they can wreak havoc on blood sugar levels. Fortunately, you have the power to outsmart them!

Practice mindful eating by paying attention to hunger and fullness cues. Plan and prepare meals in advance, so you're not caught off guard and tempted by unhealthy options when hunger strikes.

Fill your pantry with nutrient-dense snacks like nuts, seeds, and fresh fruits to satisfy cravings in a wholesome way.

*The food you eat can be either the safest and most powerful for of medicine, or the slowest form of poison.*

*Ann Wigmore*
*American Advocate*

## SUMMARY

Good job on completing this fun and informative chapter on the role of nutrition in controlling blood sugar levels! You now understand the importance of nourishing your body with real food, mindful drink choices, and wise supplementation.

By prioritising nutrition, you can empower yourself to manage blood sugar levels effectively and reduce reliance on chemical medication. Remember, healthy eating doesn't have to be boring or restrictive. Let your taste buds explore the world of nutritious and delicious options. So, get ready to savour the journey and make healthy eating your superpower in diabetes management!

Not all supplements are created equal so schedule a discovery call with us to be guided on which ones and brands we recommend. https://calendly.com/wellnessiridology

## RECOMMENDED EXERCISES :

1.WRITE DOWN AT LEAST REAL FOOD YOU WILL EAT WITH EACH MEAL TODAY.

FOR EXAMPLE, A PEAR FOR BREAKFAST, A CUCUMBER WITH LUNCH AND SOME CARROTS WITH DINNER.

....................................................................................

....................................................................................

....................................................................................

....................................................................................

....................................................................................

....................................................................................

....................................................................................

....................................................................................

....................................................................................

....................................................................................

....................................................................................

....................................................................................

....................................................................................

....................................................................................

....................................................................................

....................................................................................

2.WRITE DOWN AT LEAST ONE HEALTHY DRINK YOU WILL BE CONSUMING THROUGHOUT THE DAY.

FOR EXAMPLE, 1 LITRE OF MINERAL WATER, 1 CUP OF HERBAL TEA, 500 MLS OF COCONUT WATER.

..............................................................................

..............................................................................

..............................................................................

..............................................................................

..............................................................................

..............................................................................

..............................................................................

..............................................................................

..............................................................................

..............................................................................

..............................................................................

..............................................................................

..............................................................................

..............................................................................

..............................................................................

..............................................................................

3.WRITE DOWN AT LEAST ONE UNHEALTHY FOOD OR DRINKS INTAKE YOU WILL GIVE UP DAILY. FOR EXAMPLE, NOT EATING SWEETS AND NOT DRINKING HIGH SUGAR FIZZY DRINKS.

....................................................................................

....................................................................................

....................................................................................

....................................................................................

....................................................................................

....................................................................................

....................................................................................

....................................................................................

....................................................................................

....................................................................................

....................................................................................

....................................................................................

....................................................................................

....................................................................................

....................................................................................

....................................................................................

**NOTES :**

# *Chapter 6*

## *Making Healthier Food Choices*

*This chapter will ignite your enthusiasm for making healthier food choices!*

*Get ready to embark on a fun and encouraging journey towards a nourishing and delicious meals. In this chapter, we'll explore examples of healthier food choices and strategies to help you transition from unhealthy options.*

*Let's dive in and discover the joy of fuelling your body with wholesome goodness!*

## EMBRACE THE RAINBOW

Eating a variety of colourful fruits and vegetables is like painting your plate with vitality and nutrients. Aim to incorporate a rainbow of colours into your meals. Enjoy the sweetness of juicy berries, the crunch of vibrant bell peppers, and the earthy goodness of dark leafy greens. Experiment with different flavours, textures, and cooking methods to make your produce-packed meals exciting and enticing.

## WHOLE GRAIN WONDER

Swap refined grains for wholesome whole grains to add fibre, vitamins, and minerals to your meals. Choose options like brown rice, quinoa, spelt or rye bread, and oats. These grains provide sustained energy, promote digestive health, and keep you feeling satisfied for longer. Experiment with ancient grains like amaranth or millet to discover new and delicious alternatives.

## POWER OF PROTEIN

Protein is not only crucial for building and repairing tissues but also helps to keep you satiated. Choose lean protein sources such as skinless poultry, fish, legumes, tofu, and Greek yogurt. Explore plant-based proteins like lentils or chickpeas to add variety and flavour to your meals. Remember the importance of portion control to maintain a balanced meal.

## HEALTHY FATS FOR THE WIN

Healthy fats are good for you! Incorporate healthier sources of fats into your meals, such as avocados, nuts, seeds, and olive oil. These fats provide essential fatty acids, promote satiety, and enhance the flavours of your dishes. Whip up a delicious avocado toast, sprinkle some crushed nuts over your salads, or drizzle olive oil on roasted vegetables for a delightful and nutritious twist.

## TRANSITIONING FROM UNHEALTHY TO HEALTHY

Transitioning from unhealthy food choices can be an exciting adventure. Start by incorporating small changes gradually. For example, if you're used to sugary breakfast cereals, try swapping them for oats soaked overnight, topped with fresh fruit and a sprinkle of nuts.

Craving something crunchy? Replace potato chips with baked kale chips or roasted chickpeas. As you experience the deliciousness and benefits of healthier choices, you'll find it easier to let go of old habits.

## CELEBRATE YOUR SUCCESS

Each step towards healthier food choices is worth celebrating! Keep track of your progress and acknowledge the positive changes you've made. Share your successes with friends and family and inspire them to join you on this journey. Explore new recipes, join cooking classes, or start a healthy recipe exchange with loved ones.

Remember, healthy eating can be joyful and fulfilling!

## SUMMARY

You are doing great on embracing the exciting world of healthier food choices! By incorporating a colourful array of fruits and vegetables, whole grains, lean proteins, and healthy fats into your meals, you're fuelling your body with nourishment and vitality.

As you transition from unhealthy to healthy choices, remember to celebrate your progress and stay enthusiastic. Embrace the flavours, textures, and variety that wholesome foods offer, and invite others to join you on this delicious adventure.

Get ready to savour the joy of making healthier food choices, one tasty bite at a time!

Do check out and try our specially designed Diabetic friendly recipes below at the end of Chapter 8.

*Let food be thy medicine and medicine be thy food.*

*Hippocrates*

## RECOMMENDED EXERCISES

1. WRITE DOWN AT LEAST SIX DIFFERENT COLOURED NATURAL FOODS YOU WILL CONSUME TODAY.

FOR EXAMPLE, RED RADISHES, ORANGE CARROTS, GREEN CUCUMBER, BLUEBERRIES, PURPLE CABBAGE, YELLOW PEPPERS.

..............................................................................

..............................................................................

..............................................................................

..............................................................................

..............................................................................

..............................................................................

..............................................................................

..............................................................................

..............................................................................

..............................................................................

..............................................................................

..............................................................................

..............................................................................

..............................................................................

..............................................................................

2.WRITE DOWN AT LEAST ONE HEALTHY FAT YOU WILL BE CONSUMING TODAY.

FOR EXAMPLE, AN AVOCADO OR ADDING SOME COLD PRESSED EXTRA VIRGIN OLIVE OIL TO YOUR MEALS.

.......................................................................................

.......................................................................................

.......................................................................................

.......................................................................................

.......................................................................................

.......................................................................................

.......................................................................................

.......................................................................................

.......................................................................................

.......................................................................................

.......................................................................................

.......................................................................................

.......................................................................................

.......................................................................................

.......................................................................................

**NOTES :**

# *Chapter 7*

## *Healthy Meal Planning for Diabetes Control*

*This chapter will make healthy meal planning a breeze, even for busy individuals with packed schedules and long commutes!*

*In this easy-to-read and practical chapter, we'll explore strategies to help you plan and prepare nutritious meals that support diabetes control.*

*Get ready to discover achievable and practical tips that fit seamlessly into your busy lifestyle!*

## THE POWER OF MEAL PLANNING

Meal planning is a game-changer when it comes to eating healthy meals while managing a busy schedule. By dedicating a little time each day or week to plan your meals, you can save precious time, reduce stress, and ensure that you have balanced and diabetes-friendly options readily available.

## QUICK AND EASY MEAL PREP

For busy individuals, efficiency is key. Consider dedicating a specific day or time slot each week for meal prep. Choose recipes that are quick and easy to prepare, such as one-pan meals, sheet pan dinners, or slow cooker recipes. These options allow you to maximize your time while still enjoying nutritious and delicious meals.

Refer to our recipes in Chapter 8

## PORTABLE AND CONVENIENT OPTIONS

If you're often away from home or spend a significant amount of time commuting, it's important to have portable and convenient meal options.

Invest in leak-proof containers, reusable lunch bags, and insulated food storage to pack your meals and snacks for the day. Preparing portable meals like salads in a jar, wraps, or portioned snacks can make eating healthily on the go a breeze.

## BATCH COOKING FOR EFFICIENCY

Batch cooking is a lifesaver for busy individuals. Set aside a few hours on the weekend or a day off to cook larger quantities of staple ingredients such as grains, proteins, and roasted vegetables. Store them in individual portions, so you have the building blocks for quick and easy meals throughout the week. Utilize these pre-prepared ingredients in salads, stir-fries, or grain bowls for efficient and nutritious meals.

## HEALTHIER GRAB-AND-GO SNACKS

When hunger strikes between meals, it's important to have healthy grab-and-go snacks on hand. Stock up on portable snacks such as nuts, seeds, fresh fruit, veggie sticks with hummus, Greek yogurt cups, or homemade energy bars. These options provide a quick boost of energy without derailing your blood sugar control.

## EMBRACE TECHNOLOGY

Make use of technology to simplify your meal planning. Explore meal planning apps or websites that provide recipe suggestions, customizable meal plans, and automated grocery lists. These tools can save you time and help you stay organised, even when you're on the go.

## SUMMARY

Bravo on discovering the secrets of healthy meal planning for diabetes control! By incorporating efficient strategies like meal prep, batch cooking, and embracing portable options, you can easily maintain a balanced and nutritious meals despite your busy schedule and commuting demands.

Remember to prioritise your health and well-being by making time for meal planning and preparation. With a little organization and the right tools, you'll be equipped to enjoy diabetes-friendly meals that support your blood sugar control, no matter how busy life gets.

So, get ready to conquer your schedule with practical and achievable healthy meal planning strategies!

**NOTES :**

**YOU ARE A QUARTER WAY INTO THIS BOOK. KEEP GOING!**

**NOTES :**

..........................................................................................................
..........................................................................................................
..........................................................................................................
..........................................................................................................
..........................................................................................................
..........................................................................................................
..........................................................................................................
..........................................................................................................
..........................................................................................................
..........................................................................................................
..........................................................................................................
..........................................................................................................
..........................................................................................................
..........................................................................................................
..........................................................................................................
..........................................................................................................
..........................................................................................................
..........................................................................................................
..........................................................................................................
..........................................................................................................
..........................................................................................................
..........................................................................................................
..........................................................................................................
..........................................................................................................
..........................................................................................................
..........................................................................................................

**YOU ARE A QUARTER WAY INTO THIS BOOK. KEEP GOING!**

# *Chapter 8*

## *Cooking Methods & Recipes for Blood Sugar*

*Welcome to the exciting world of cooking methods and recipes that support healthy blood sugar levels!*

*In this fun and practical chapter, we'll explore the use of good quality cooking oils, cookware, and share several delightful recipes that can be prepared within minutes.*

*Get ready to infuse your culinary adventures with deliciousness and blood sugar-friendly goodness!*

## CHOOSING GOOD QUALITY COOKING OILS

When it comes to cooking, choosing the right oils is essential. Choose good quality, heart-healthy cooking oils such as olive oil, avocado oil, or coconut oil. These oils contain beneficial fats and are less likely to cause spikes in blood sugar.

Experiment with different oils to discover flavours that complement your recipes and elevate your culinary creations.

## COOKWARE FOR HEALTHY MEALS

Cooking with the right cookware can make a difference in your blood sugar control. Invest in good quality cookware that does not contain aluminium or other chemicals that may leech into your food when cooking on high heat or when the cookware is scratched over time. Additionally, consider using oven-safe containers for roasting vegetables or baking lean proteins, as this method requires minimal oil while keeping the flavours ntact.

*Chapter 8*

# QUICK AND DELICIOUS RECIPES

Let's dive into some blood sugar-friendly recipes that can be prepared within minutes.

## 1.PROTEIN AND VEGGIE STIR-FRY

Ingredients:

Assorted vegetables (such as bell peppers, broccoli, carrots, snap peas)

Lean protein of your choice (tofu, shrimp, chicken breast)

Sea salt

1 to 2 cloves minced garlic.

1 to 2 shallots finely diced.

1 thumb size grated ginger with the skin

1 tablespoon Sesame oil (optional)

Instructions:

Heat a pan or wok over medium-high heat and add a small amount of olive or coconut oil.

Add minced garlic, diced shallots and grated ginger, and stir-fry for a minute until fragrant.

Add your choice of lean protein. Stir-fry for a few minutes and then add in the vegetables of your choice. Ensure the vegetables remain tender-crisp and the protein is cooked through.

Sprinkle some sea salt per your taste and toss to mix evenly. Optional: Add a splash of sesame oil for extra flavour. Serve hot and enjoy!

# Protein and Veggie Stir-Fry

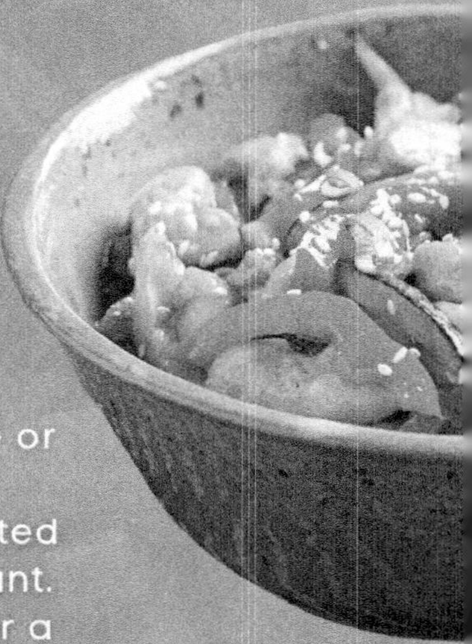

**Ingredients:**

-Assorted vegetables (such as bell peppers, broccoli, carrots, snap peas)
-Lean protein of your choice (tofu, shrimp, chicken breast)
-Sea salt
-1 to 2 cloves minced garlic
-1 to 2 shallots finely diced
-1 thumb size grated ginger with the skin
-1 tablespoon Sesame oil (optional)

**Instructions:**

-Heat a pan or wok over medium
-high heat and add a small amount of olive or coconut oil.
-Add minced garlic, diced shallots and grated ginger, and stir-fry for a minute until fragrant.
-Add your choice of lean protein. Stir-fry for a few minutes and then add in the vegetables of your choice.
-Ensure the vegetables remain tender-crisp and the protein is cooked through.
-Sprinkle some sea salt per your taste and toss to mix evenly.

*Optional: Add a splash of sesame oil for extra flavour. *Serve hot and enjoy!

## 2.QUINOA SALAD

Ingredients:

Cooked quinoa
Assorted chopped vegetables such as cucumber, cherry tomatoes, red onion.
Fresh herbs such as parsley, mint, or basil
Lemon juice
Extra virgin olive oil
Sea salt per taste

Instructions:

In a bowl, combine cooked quiroa, chopped vegetables, and fresh herbs.
Drizzle with lemon juice and extra virg n olive oil.
Season with sea salt and toss to combine.
Let the flavours marinate for a few minutes.
Serve chilled or at room temperature as a refreshing and nutritious salad.

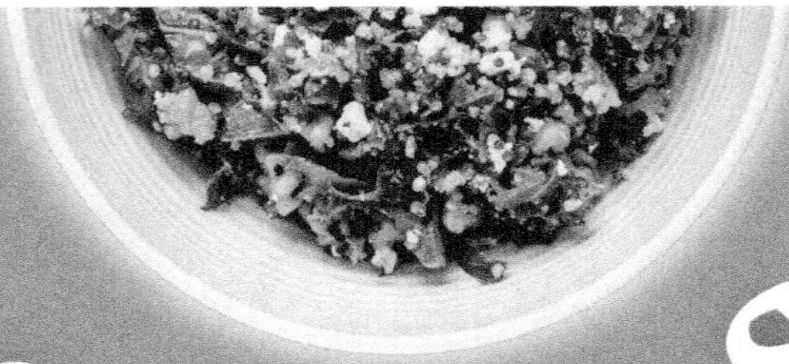

# Quinoa Salad

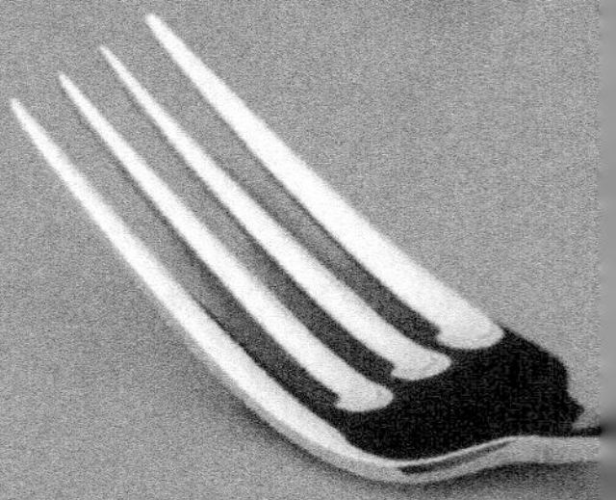

## Ingredients:

-Cooked quinoa
-Assorted chopped vegetables such as cucumber, cherry tomatoes, red onion
-Fresh herbs such as parsley, mint, or basil
-Lemon juice
-Extra virgin olive oil
-Sea salt per taste

## Instructions:

-In a bowl, combine cooked quinoa, chopped vegetables, and fresh herbs.
-Drizzle with lemon juice and extra virgin olive oil.
-Season with sea salt and toss to combine.
Let the flavours marinate for a few minutes.

*Serve chilled or at room temperature as a refreshing and nutritious salad.

PLANET WELLNESS

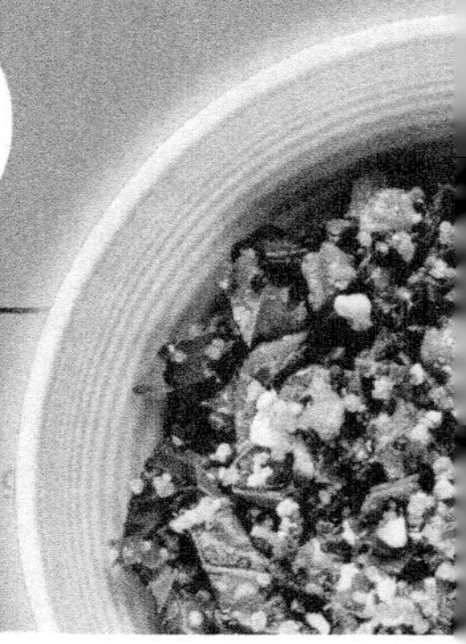

@planetwellness
@planetwellness
@planetwellness
@planetwellnessiridolo

### 3.BAKED SALMON

Ingredients:

Salmon fillets
Lemon slices
Fresh dill or your preferred herbs

Instructions:

Preheat the oven to 375°F (190°C) and line a baking sheet with parchment paper.
Place the salmon fillets on the prepared baking sheet.
Season with salt and your choice of herbs.
Top each fillet with a lemon slice for added flavour.
Bake for approximately 12-15 minutes or until the salmon is cooked to your desired doneness.
Serve hot and enjoy the succulent flavours of baked salmon.

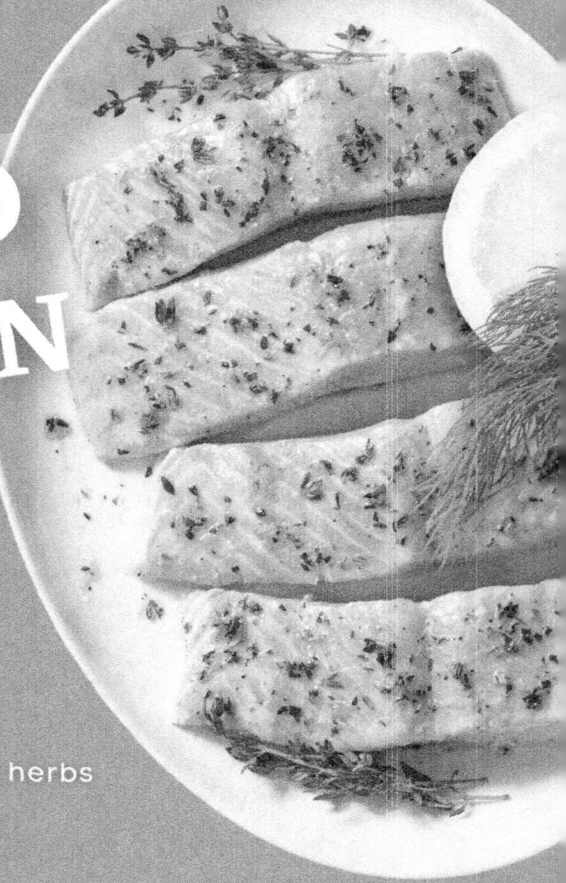

# BAKED SALMON

## Ingredients:

-Salmon fillets
-Lemon slices
-Fresh dill or your preferred herbs

## Instructions:

-Preheat the oven to 375°F (190°C) and line a baking sheet with parchment paper.
-Place the salmon fillets on the prepared baking sheet.
-Season with salt and your choice of herbs.
-Top each fillet with a lemon slice for added flavour.
-Bake for approximately 12-15 minutes or until the salmon is cooked to your desired doneness.

*Serve hot and enjoy the succulent flavours of baked salmon.

## 4.BITTER GOURD RECIPE

This vegetable is renowned for managing or reversing Diabetes. It may take a bit of getting used to due to its bitter taste.

Ingredients:
1 bitter gourd
1 shallot and other vegetables such as carrots (optional)
Sea salt and herbs such as coriander or chives

Instructions:

Boil some water in a steamer.
Whilst waiting for the water to boil, wash and cut the bitter gourd into bite size pieces.
Add the cut pieces to the steamer and steam for maximum 5 minutes. The bitter gourd should still retain its colour and crunchy.
Remove from heat and serve with sea salt and herbs.

*Bitter Gourd / Foo Kua / Bitter Melon / Karela / Corilla/Margoze / Momordica Charantia*

# Cooking Instructions

- Wash the bitter gourd thoroughly with bio degradable detergent.
- Brush it well to remove all dirt/toxins.
- Then follow the following cooking instructions:

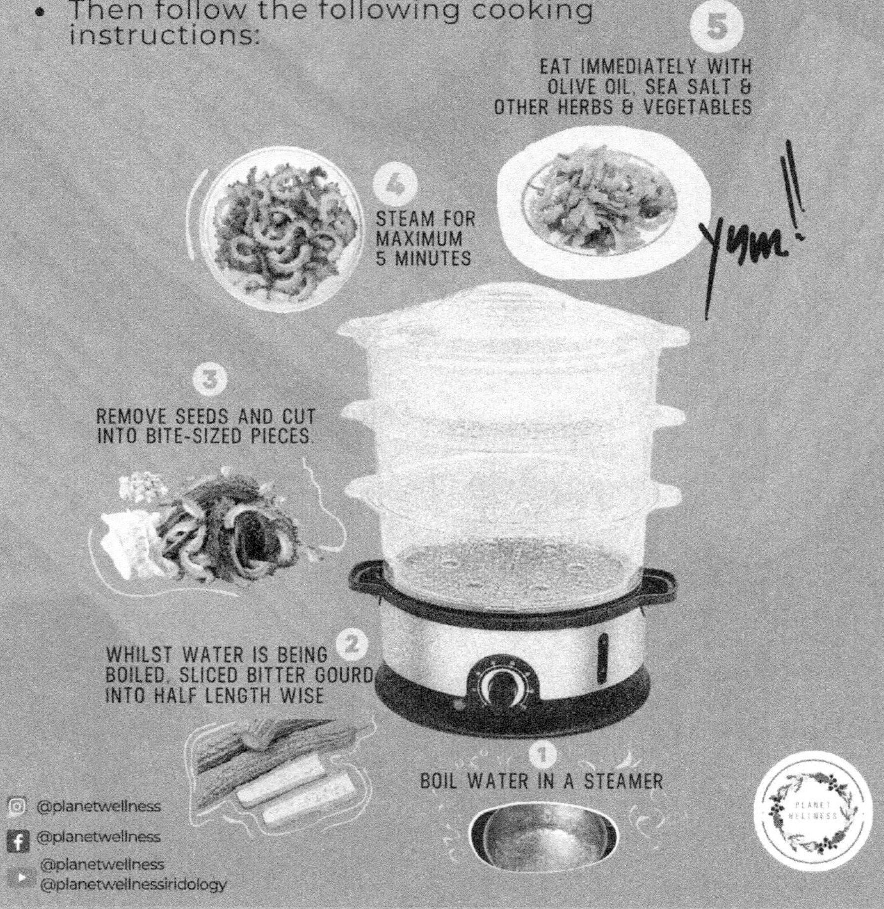

## 5.SWEET POTATO AND PONTIAC POTATO VEGETARIAN OR FISH CAKES

Ingredients:

1 medium or large, sweet potato
2 medium Pontiac potatoes
1 shallot
1 carrot
100 grams garden peas
1 tablespoon turmeric
Sea salt and herbs such as coriander or chives
2 tablespoons spelt flour
1 can sardines or red salmon (fish cake option)

Instructions:

Wash, finely dice and steam for at least 5 minutes, the sweet potato and Pontiac potatoes with the skin on.

Whilst waiting for the potatoes to be cooked, finely dice the shallot and carrots.

Remove the potatoes from the steamer and place in a bowl.

Mash the potatoes and mix in the turmeric, sea salt, herbs, garden peas, shallot, carrot, spelt flour and fish.

Preheat the oven to 375°F (190°C) and line a baking sheet with parchment paper.

Shape into cake size of your choice and bake for at least 10 minutes, turning the cake over after few minutes.
Alternatively, you can shallow fry the cakes with olive oil.

Serve hot and enjoy!

# Sweet Potato and Pontiac Potato Vegetarian or Fish Cakes

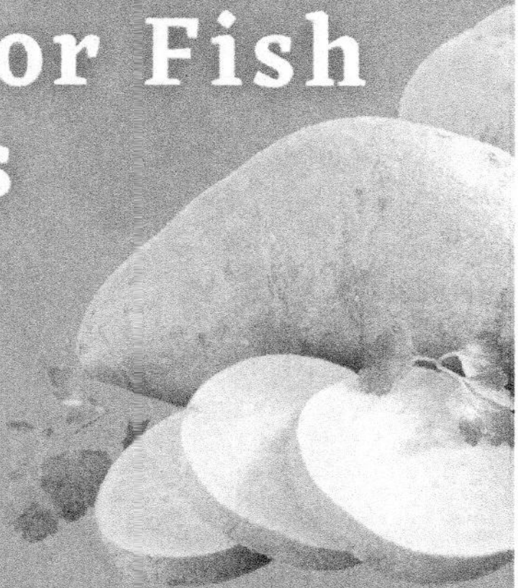

**Ingredients:**

-1 medium or large, sweet potato
-2 medium Pontiac potatoes
-1 shallot
-1 carrot
-100 grams garden peas
-1 tablespoon turmeric
-Sea salt and herbs such as coriander or chives
-2 tablespoons spelt flour
-1 can sardines or red salmon (fish cake option)

**Instructions:**

-Wash, finely dice and steam for at least 5 minutes, the sweet potato and Pontiac potatoes with the skin on.
-Whilst waiting for the potatoes to be cooked, finely dice the shallot and carrots.
-Remove the potatoes from the steamer and place in a bowl.
-Mash the potatoes and mix in the turmeric, sea salt, herbs, garden peas, shallot, carrot, spelt flour and fish.
-Preheat the oven to 375°F (190°C) and line a baking sheet with parchment paper.
-Shape into cake size of your choice and bake for at least 10 minutes, turning the cake over after few minutes.
*Alternatively, you can shallow fry the cakes with olive oil. Serve hot and enjoy!

PLANET WELLNESS

@planetwellness
@planetwellness
@planetwellness
@planetwellnessiridology

## 6.BROWN, RED AND WILD RICE

Most people have been accustomed to eating white rice and have it in their minds that the curry and other dishes taste better with the white rice. Although it does not taste sweet, research has proven that white rice contains more sugar than glucose. White rice is therefore one of the leading causes of Diabetes worldwide.

Our recipe of mixed rice is much healthier, and we have proven over the years that when you keep an open mind, you will enjoy this rice dish going forward.

Ingredients:
40 grams brown rice
40 grams red rice
20 grams wild rice
1 shallot
1 red onion
1 thumb size ginger with the skin
Vegetables such as carrots, eggplant and peas
Sea salt per taste

Instructions:

Wash the rice mixture and add to a pot with at least 2x the quantity of water to rice. Bring to boil on low heat.

In the meantime, finely dice the shallots, onions, ginger and vegetables of your choice.

When rice is almost cooked, stir in the finely diced ingredients and cook for at least 5 minutes.

Serve with olive oil, herbs such as coriander and chives.

Enjoy with a rainbow salad or other cooked dishes.

# BROWN, RED AND WILD RICE

**Ingredients:**

- -40 grams Brown Rice
- -40 grams Red Rice
- -20 grams Wild Rice
- -1 Shallot
- -1 Red Onion
- -1 Thumb size ginger with the skin
- -Vegetables such as carrots, eggplant and peas
- -Sea salt per taste

**Instructions:**

-Wash the rice mixture and add to a pot with at least 2x the quantity of water to rice.
-Bring to boil on low heat.
-In the meantime, finely dice the shallots, onions, ginger and vegetables of your choice.
-When rice is almost cooked, stir in the finely diced ingredients and cook for at least 5 minutes.
-Serve with olive oil, herbs such as coriander and chives.
-Enjoy with a rainbow salad or other cooked dishes.

PLANET WELLNESS

@planetwellness
@planetwellness
@planetwellness
@planetwellnessiridology

## SUMMARY

Well done on exploring cooking methods and recipes that support healthy blood sugar levels.

By using good quality cooking oils, choosing appropriate cookware, and trying out delicious recipes like veggie stir-fry, quinoa salad, and baked salmon, you can enjoy meals that are both quick and blood sugar friendly.

Remember to have fun in the kitchen, experiment with flavours, and savour the joy of creating nutritious meals.

So, grab your apron, preheat the stove, and get ready to indulge in tasty, diabetes-friendly delights!

## NOTES :

# *Chapter 9*

## *The Benefits of Fibre-Rich Foods for Blood Sugar Control*

*Welcome to the chapter that celebrates your progress and highlights the incredible benefits of fibre-rich foods for blood sugar control!*

*In this easy-to-read chapter, we'll explore the power of fibre and provide examples of fibre-rich foods that can support your journey towards optimal blood sugar levels.*

*Let's dive in and discover the remarkable benefits of incorporating fibre into your meals.*

*Chapter 9*

## THE MARVELS OF FIBRE

Fibre is like a superhero for blood sugar control. It slows down the digestion and absorption of carbohydrates, preventing rapid spikes in blood sugar levels. Additionally, fibre promotes feelings of fullness, helps regulate bowel movements, and supports overall digestive health. By embracing fibre-rich foods, you're empowering yourself to manage blood sugar effectively and enhance your overall well-being.

## EXAMPLES OF FIBRE-RICH FOODS

To reap the benefits of fibre, incorporate a variety of fibre-rich foods into your meals. Here are some examples of delicious options:

Whole grains: Quinoa, brown rice, oats, whole wheat bread, and barley.

Legumes: Lentils, chickpeas, black beans, and kidney beans.

Fruits: Berries, apples, pears, oranges, and avocados.

Vegetables: Broccoli, Brussels sprouts, carrots, spinach, and kale.

Nuts and seeds: Almonds, chia seeds, flaxseeds, and walnuts.

These are just a few examples. The world of fibre-rich foods is vast and exciting. Explore different options, experiment with new recipes, and savour the diverse flavours and textures that fibre-rich foods have to offer.

## CELEBRATING YOUR PROGRESS

As you reach the end of this chapter, take a moment to reflect on the knowledge you've gained about the benefits of fibre for blood sugar control. You've taken an important step towards understanding the role of fibre in your meals and its impact on your overall health. By incorporating fibre-rich foods into your meals, you're making a positive and impactful choice for your well-being.

## SUMMARY

You've completed this chapter on the benefits of fibre-rich foods for blood sugar control, and that's something to be proud of! By embracing fibre, you're harnessing the power of slow digestion, improved satiety, and enhanced digestive health.

Remember to include a variety of fibre-rich foods in your meals, such as whole grains, legumes, fruits, vegetables, nuts, and seeds. These choices will not only support your blood sugar control but also provide a myriad of other health benefits.

So, give yourself a pat on the back for completing this chapter and continue your journey towards optimal health and blood sugar control!

**NOTES :**

..........................................................................................
..........................................................................................
..........................................................................................
..........................................................................................
..........................................................................................
..........................................................................................
..........................................................................................
..........................................................................................
..........................................................................................
..........................................................................................
..........................................................................................
..........................................................................................
..........................................................................................
..........................................................................................
..........................................................................................
..........................................................................................
..........................................................................................
..........................................................................................
..........................................................................................
..........................................................................................

# *Chapter 10*

## *The Role of Protein and Healthy Fats in Diabetes Management*

*This chapter unveils the importance of protein and healthy fats in diabetes management.*

*In this easy-to-read chapter, we'll explore the significant role that protein and healthy fats play in supporting your blood sugar control.*

*Whether you follow a vegetarian, vegan, or food choices, we've got you covered with a range of examples that cater to diverse meal preferences.*

*Let's dive in and discover the power of protein and healthy fats for diabetes management!*

Protein is an essential nutrient that plays a vital role in diabetes management. It helps to stabilize blood sugar levels, promote feelings of fullness, and support muscle maintenance and repair. Include a variety of protein sources in your diet to ensure you meet your nutritional needs.

Here are some examples of healthy protein options:

Lean meats: Skinless poultry, turkey, and lean cuts of beef.

Fish: Salmon, tuna, mackerel, and sardines, which are also rich in heart-healthy omega-3 fatty acids.

Legumes: Lentils, chickpeas, black beans, and tofu (for vegetarian and vegan options).

Dairy and dairy alternatives: Greek yogurt, cottage cheese, and almond milk or soy milk fortified with protein.

Eggs: A versatile and protein-packed option that can be enjoyed in various ways.

## EMBRACING HEALTHY FATS

Healthy fats are an essential part of a balanced meal and are beneficial for blood sugar control. They provide energy, support nutrient absorption, and contribute to overall satiety. Choose sources of healthy fats to enhance your diabetes management.

Below are some examples of healthy fat options:

Avocados: A creamy and nutritious fruit rich in monounsaturated fats.

Nuts and seeds: Almonds, walnuts, chia seeds, flaxseeds, sunflower seeds and pumpkin seeds.
Olive oil: A heart-healthy oil that can be used for cooking and dressing salads.

Fatty fish: Salmon, trout, and sardines, which are also excellent sources of omega-3 fatty acids.

Coconut and coconut oil: A versatile option that can add a touch of flavour to various dishes.

## PLANT-BASED PROTEIN SOURCES

For those following a vegetarian, vegan, or plant-based lifestyle, there are plenty of protein-rich options available. These alternatives not only provide protein but also offer a range of other beneficial nutrients.

Here are some plant-based protein sources to consider:

Legumes and pulses: Lentils, chickpeas, black beans, and edamame.

Tofu and tempeh: Versatile soy-based options that can be incorporated into various recipes.

Quinoa and other ancient grains: Complete protein sources that provide a range of essential nutrients.

Nut and seed butters: Almond butter, Hazelnut butter and tahini.

Plant-based protein powders: Pea protein, brown rice protein, and hemp protein.

## SUMMARY

You've reached the end of this chapter on the role of protein and healthy fats in diabetes management. By incorporating healthy protein and fat sources into your meals, you're supporting blood sugar control, promoting satiety, and nourishing your body with essential nutrients.

Whether you prefer lean meats, fish, legumes, plant-based options, or a combination of choices, there are numerous possibilities to cater to your dietary preferences and lifestyle.

So, embrace the power of protein and healthy fats as you continue your journey towards optimal diabetes management and overall well-being!

## NOTES :

................................................................................

................................................................................

................................................................................

................................................................................

................................................................................

................................................................................

................................................................................

................................................................................

................................................................................

................................................................................

................................................................................

................................................................................

................................................................................

................................................................................

................................................................................

................................................................................

................................................................................

................................................................................

................................................................................

................................................................................

**NOTES :**

.......................................................................................

.......................................................................................

.......................................................................................

.......................................................................................

.......................................................................................

.......................................................................................

.......................................................................................

.......................................................................................

.......................................................................................

.......................................................................................

.......................................................................................

.......................................................................................

.......................................................................................

.......................................................................................

.......................................................................................

.......................................................................................

.......................................................................................

.......................................................................................

.......................................................................................

.......................................................................................

# *Chapter 11*

## *Mindful Eating: Developing a Healthy Relationship with Food*

*This chapter will revolutionise your relationship with food and empower you to become a mindful eater!*

*In this enticing chapter, we'll explore strategies to help even the fussiest eaters and those with ingrained poor food choices develop a healthier mindset towards eating.*

*We'll also delve into tips for weaning off unhealthier foods and managing comfort and binge eating.*

*Get ready to embark on a transformative journey towards mindful eating and a positive relationship with food!*

## EMBRACING MINDFUL EATING

Mindful eating is about more than just what you eat. It's about how you eat. By practicing mindful eating, you cultivate awareness, attentiveness, and gratitude for the food you consume. It involves paying attention to your body's hunger and fullness cues, savouring each bite, and honouring the nourishment that food provides. Mindful eating can help shift your perspective and create a healthier relationship with food.

## OVERCOMING FUSSY EATING

If you're a fussy eater, expanding your food choices can be a gradual and enjoyable process. Start by introducing small changes and experimenting with new flavours and textures. Try incorporating new foods into dishes you already enjoy, such as adding vegetables to a stir-fry or blending fruits into a smoothie. Approach new foods with curiosity and an open mind, allowing yourself to discover a wider range of options that can contribute to your health and well-being.

## TRANSFORMING POOR FOOD CHOICES

If your food choices have been influenced by upbringing or cultural practices that prioritize less healthy options, transforming those habits may require a conscious effort. Start by educating yourself about the benefits of nutritious foods and the impact they can have on your overall health.

Gradually introduce healthier alternatives while still honouring your cultural background. Seek out recipes and cooking techniques that retain the flavours and traditions you cherish, but with a healthier twist. It's about finding a balance that aligns with your goals while staying connected to your roots.

## WEANING OFF UNHEALTHIER FOODS

Weaning off unhealthier foods can be a gradual process that involves replacing them with more nutritious options. Begin by identifying the unhealthier foods that you frequently consume and find healthier alternatives that provide similar satisfaction.

For example, swap sugary drinks for flavoured water or herbal teas, replace processed snacks with fresh fruit or homemade energy bars, and choose whole grains over refined grains. Be patient and kind to yourself during this transition, celebrating each small step towards healthier choices.

## MANAGING COMFORT AND BINGE EATING

Comfort and binge eating can pose challenges when it comes to developing a healthy relationship with food. Start by understanding the triggers and emotions that lead to these behaviours

Instead of turning to food for comfort, explore alternative coping mechanisms such as engaging in physical activity, journaling, talking to a supportive friend, or practicing relaxation techniques.

Seek professional help if needed, as a therapist or counsellor can provide guidance and support to address emotional eating patterns.

## SUMMARY

Congratulations on reaching the end of this transformative chapter on mindful eating and developing a healthy relationship with food! By embracing mindful eating, you can shift your perspective, overcome fussy eating habits, and transform ingrained poor food choices.

Remember to approach changes gradually, celebrate small victories, and be kind to yourself throughout the journey. By practicing mindful eating, you can savour the joy of nourishing your body, honour your cultural background, and discover a newfound appreciation for a wide range of healthier options.

So, let go of judgment, embrace curiosity, and embark on the path to mindful eating and a positive relationship with food!

“

*Food is the most abused anxiety drug.*

*Exercise is the most underutilised antidepressant.*

”

**NOTES :**

# *Chapter 12*

## *Strategies for Dining Out with Diabetes*

*In this chapter, we will make dining out with diabetes a fun and practical experience!*

*We will explore strategies to help you navigate social gatherings, make healthier choices, and strike a balance between enjoying your meal and managing your blood sugar levels.*

*Get ready to embark on a journey filled with delicious and mindful dining!*

*Chapter 12*

## EMBRACE THE ADVENTURE

Dining out should be an enjoyable experience, even with diabetes. Approach it as an adventure to try new flavours, savour the company of friends and loved ones, and celebrate good food.

By adopting a positive mindset, you can navigate menus and make healthier choices without feeling deprived.

## PLAN

Before heading to a restaurant, take a moment to review the menu online, if available. Look for healthier options that align with your meal choices, such as grilled or baked proteins, vegetable-based dishes, and whole grain options.

Planning can help you make informed choices and prevent impulse decisions at the table.

## CHOOSE BALANCED MEALS

When dining out, aim for balanced meals that include a combination of lean protein, fibre-rich carbohydrates, and healthy fats. Choose grilled or baked proteins like fish or chicken, go for whole grain options like brown rice or whole wheat bread, and incorporate plenty of vegetables into your meal. This balance helps manage blood sugar levels and provides essential nutrients.

## BE MINDFUL OF PORTIONS

Restaurant portions are often larger than what we need. Be mindful of portion sizes and consider sharing a dish with a friend or asking for a take-out container to save leftovers. Alternatively, you can order an appetizer or choose smaller plate options if available.

Remember, it's not only about what you eat but also how much you eat.

## CUSTOMISE YOUR ORDER

Be bold and request to customise your order to fit your meal choices. Ask for sauces, dressings, or gravies on the side so you can control the amount you consume. Request steamed or grilled preparations instead of fried options. Most restaurants are accommodating and willing to adjust meet your preferences.

## BE SOCIABLE AND MAKE HEALTHIER CHOICES

Eating out doesn't mean you have to sacrifice socialising. Engage in conversations, enjoy the ambiance, and make healthier choices simultaneously. Instead of calorie-laden drinks, opt for sparkling water with a slice of lemon or lime.

Choose fresh salads as a starter or side dish. If dessert is a must, consider sharing it with others to satisfy your sweet tooth without overindulging.

## KNOW YOUR LIMITS

While it's essential to enjoy dining out, it's also important to know your limits. Be mindful of portion sizes, added sugars, and unhealthy fats. It's perfectly okay to indulge occasionally but be aware of your overall meal goals and draw the line when necessary. Strive for a balance between enjoying yourself and taking care of your health.

## SUMMARY

Congratulations on discovering strategies for dining out with diabetes! By embracing the adventure, planning, opting for balanced meals, being mindful of portions, customising your order, and knowing your limits, you can navigate social gatherings while making healthier choices. Remember, it's not about being 100% strict with your choices every day but rather finding a balance that supports your overall well-being. So, embark on your next dining out experience with confidence, knowing that you can enjoy good food, great company, and make choices that align with your health goals. Bon appétit!

**NOTES :**

....................................................................................................

....................................................................................................

....................................................................................................

....................................................................................................

....................................................................................................

....................................................................................................

....................................................................................................

....................................................................................................

....................................................................................................

....................................................................................................

....................................................................................................

....................................................................................................

....................................................................................................

....................................................................................................

....................................................................................................

....................................................................................................

....................................................................................................

....................................................................................................

....................................................................................................

....................................................................................................

**NOTES :**

# *Chapter 13*

## *Dealing with Food Cravings & Emotional Eating*

*This chapter will equip you with practical strategies to overcome food cravings and emotional eating, particularly when it comes to highly processed foods containing white sugar and white rice.*

*In this chapter, we'll explore methods to address cravings, distinguish physical hunger from emotional hunger, and provide actionable tips to curb emotional eating.*

*Get ready to regain control and foster a healthier relationship with food!*

*Chapter 13*

## UNDERSTANDING FOOD CRAVINGS

Food cravings can be powerful and challenging to resist, especially when it comes to highly processed foods that contain white sugar and white rice. These foods can create addictive-like responses in the brain, leading to intense cravings. Recognizing this is the first step towards managing cravings effectively.

### Distinguishing Physical Hunger from Emotional Hunger:

It's important to differentiate between physical hunger and emotional hunger. Physical hunger arises gradually and is accompanied by physical cues such as a growling stomach or feelings of light-headedness. Emotional hunger, on the other hand, is often sudden, intense, and driven by specific emotions. By becoming aware of these differences, you can address your cravings more effectively.

## PRACTICAL STRATEGIES TO CURB CRAVINGS

1.Choose nutrient-dense alternatives:

When a craving strikes, reach for healthier alternatives that satisfy both your taste buds and nutritional needs. For instance, replace sugary desserts with a piece of fresh fruit or a small serving of Greek yogurt topped with berries and a sprinkle of nuts.

2.Sip on herbal tea or flavoured water:

Sometimes, cravings can be alleviated by drinking something flavourful without the added sugars. Sip on herbal tea or infuse your water with slices of citrus fruits or cucumber to satisfy your craving for a refreshing beverage.

3.Practice mindful eating:

Slow down and savour each bite, paying attention to the flavours, textures, and sensations of the food.

Engaging in mindful eating can help you become more attuned to your body's signals of fullness and satisfaction, reducing the intensity of cravings.

4. Address underlying emotional needs:

Cravings can often be triggered by emotional states. Instead of turning to food as a coping mechanism, explore alternative ways to address and process your emotions. Engage in activities that bring you joy, such as going for a walk, dancing, journaling, or talking to a supportive friend.

## COPING WITH EMOTIONAL EATING

1. Recognise emotional triggers: Be mindful of the emotions that may lead to emotional eating. Awareness is key to breaking the cycle. Pay attention to times when you're more prone to emotional eating, such as when stressed, bored, or lonely.

2. Find healthy outlets: Discover alternative ways to cope with emotions that don't involve food. Engage in activities that bring you joy, such as exercising, practicing mindfulness or deep breathing exercises, engaging in hobbies, or seeking support from loved ones.

3. Create a supportive environment: Stock your pantry and refrigerator with healthier options to reduce the temptation of highly processed foods. Surround yourself with positive influences that encourage healthier habits and reinforce your commitment to managing emotional eating.

*Chapter 13*

## SUMMARY

Congratulations on exploring strategies to overcome food cravings and emotional eating, particularly when it comes to highly processed foods containing white sugar and white rice!

By recognizing the differences between physical and emotional hunger, opting for healthier alternatives, practicing mindful eating, and finding healthier outlets for emotional needs, you can regain control and develop a healthier relationship with food.

Remember, it's a journey that requires self-compassion and patience. By implementing these practical tips, you'll be well-equipped to address cravings and manage emotional eating, fostering a balanced and nourishing approach to your overall well-being.

**NOTES :**

.............................................................................................................

.............................................................................................................

.............................................................................................................

.............................................................................................................

.............................................................................................................

.............................................................................................................

.............................................................................................................

.............................................................................................................

.............................................................................................................

.............................................................................................................

.............................................................................................................

.............................................................................................................

.............................................................................................................

.............................................................................................................

.............................................................................................................

.............................................................................................................

.............................................................................................................

.............................................................................................................

.............................................................................................................

.............................................................................................................

# *Chapter 14*

## *Tracking & Monitoring Blood Sugar Levels*

*This chapter will guide you through the process of tracking and monitoring your blood sugar levels.*

*In this easy-to-read and practical chapter, we'll explore simple yet effective methods to help you stay on top of your diabetes management.*

*Get ready to take charge of your health and gain valuable insights into your blood sugar control!*

*Chapter 14*

## THE IMPORTANCE OF TRACKING

Tracking your blood sugar levels is a crucial aspect of diabetes management. It allows you to monitor how your body responds to various foods, activities, and medications. By keeping a record of your blood sugar readings, you can identify patterns, make informed decisions, and work towards optimal control.

Choose a Tracking Method that Works for You.

There are several ways to track and monitor your blood sugar levels, so choose a method that suits your lifestyle and preferences:

Traditional Logbook:

Keep a paper logbook to jot down your blood sugar readings, along with notes on meals, exercise, and any other relevant information. This method is straightforward and accessible, requiring only a pen and paper.

Smartphone Apps:

Use diabetes management apps on your smartphone to track blood sugar levels digitally. These apps often come with additional features like tracking medication, meal intake, and exercise, making it convenient to have all your data in one place.

Glucose Meters with Memory Function:

If your glucose meter has a memory function, take advantage of it to store your readings. This can be useful for reviewing trends and patterns over time.

Tracking Tips for Practicality:

To make tracking and monitoring blood sugar levels more practical, consider the following tips:

Set Reminders:
Use alarms or smartphone notifications to remind you to check your blood sugar levels at specific times throughout the day. Consistency is key in maintaining an accurate record.

Be Mindful of Timing:
Record the time of day when you check your blood sugar levels, as it can provide valuable information about your body's response to meals and activities.

Note Additional Factors:
Alongside your blood sugar readings, make notes of factors that may impact your levels, such as stress, illness, medication changes, or significant lifestyle events. These details can help you identify potential triggers or trends in your blood sugar control.

Regular Review and Evaluation:
Regularly review and evaluate your blood sugar tracking data to identify patterns, trends, and potential areas for improvement. Consider sharing this information with your healthcare team during check-ups to gain insights and collaborate on your diabetes management plan.

Celebrate Progress and Stay Motivated:
Recognize and celebrate the progress you make in managing your blood sugar levels.

Even small improvements and maintaining consistent control are worth acknowledging. Use these achievements as motivation to continue taking charge of your health.

## SUMMARY

Congratulations on learning the importance of tracking and monitoring your blood sugar levels! By choosing a tracking method that works for you, being consistent in your efforts, and regularly reviewing your data, you are taking proactive steps towards better diabetes management.

Remember, tracking is not only about recording numbers but also gaining valuable insights into your body's response to various factors. Stay motivated, celebrate your progress, and continue working with your healthcare team to achieve optimal blood sugar control. With these practical tracking strategies, you're well-equipped to navigate your diabetes journey with confidence and empowerment.

Amazing. You are halfway through this book. Keep up the great progress.

**NOTES :**

........................................................................................

........................................................................................

........................................................................................

........................................................................................

........................................................................................

........................................................................................

........................................................................................

........................................................................................

........................................................................................

........................................................................................

........................................................................................

........................................................................................

........................................................................................

........................................................................................

........................................................................................

........................................................................................

........................................................................................

........................................................................................

........................................................................................

........................................................................................

**NOTES :**

......................................................................................

......................................................................................

......................................................................................

......................................................................................

......................................................................................

......................................................................................

......................................................................................

......................................................................................

......................................................................................

......................................................................................

......................................................................................

......................................................................................

......................................................................................

......................................................................................

......................................................................................

......................................................................................

......................................................................................

......................................................................................

......................................................................................

......................................................................................

# *Chapter 15*

## *Visualisation, Positive Thinking & Healing*

*This chapter will introduce you to the transformative power of visualisation, positive thinking, and healing.*

*In this chapter, we'll explore practical examples and the best approaches for those who are new to these practices.*

*Get ready to tap into your inner strength and harness the incredible potential of your mind for healing and well-being!*

*Chapter 15*

## THE POWER OF VISUALISATION

Visualisation is a technique that involves creating vivid mental images of desired outcomes or experiences. It harnesses the power of your imagination to positively influence your thoughts, emotions, and actions.

Below is a practical approach to incorporating visualisation into your life:

·Find a quiet and comfortable space where you won't be disturbed.

·Close your eyes and take a few deep breaths to relax your mind and body.

·Imagine yourself in a specific situation or achieving a particular goal related to your health and well-being.

·Engage your senses by visualising the details: Colours, textures, sounds, and even the emotions associated with the experience.

·Hold onto that image and let yourself feel the joy, confidence, and positive energy it brings.

·Repeat this visualisation practice regularly to reinforce positive thoughts and beliefs.

## CULTIVATING POSITIVE THINKING

Positive thinking involves consciously choosing to focus on the positive aspects of life, fostering a mindset of optimism and gratitude.

Here are practical ways to cultivate positive thinking:

·Start your day with positive affirmations. Repeat empowering statements such as "I am capable," "I am resilient," or "I am in control of my health."

·Surround yourself with positive influences. Engage in activities, read books, or listen to podcasts that inspire and uplift you.

·Practice gratitude by reflecting on and appreciating the blessings in your life. Keep a gratitude journal to jot down things you're thankful for each day.

·Challenge negative thoughts and reframe them with positive alternatives. Instead of dwelling on what went wrong, focus on what you learned or how you can grow from the experience.

## Chapter 15

### HEALING THROUGH MIND-BODY CONNECTION:

The mind-body connection acknowledges the influence our thoughts, emotions, and beliefs have on our physical health.

Here's a practical approach to promote healing through the mind-body connection:

·Practice mindfulness. Set aside dedicated time each day to quiet your mind, focus on your breath, and cultivate awareness of the present moment.

·Engage in relaxation techniques, such as deep breathing exercises, progressive muscle relaxation, or guided imagery, to promote physical and mental relaxation.

·Incorporate activities that bring you joy and promote a sense of well-being, such as engaging in hobbies, spending time in nature, or listening to soothing music.

·Seek support from others who understand and support your healing journey, such as joining support groups, seeking therapy, or connecting with like-minded individuals.

## EMBRACING THE LEARNING PROCESS

Remember, these practices may be new to you, and it takes time and patience to fully integrate them into your life. Embrace the learning process and be gentle with yourself along the way. Each step you take towards visualisation, positive thinking, and healing contributes to your overall well-being.

## SUMMARY

Well done on exploring the transformative practices of visualisation, positive thinking, and healing! By incorporating visualisation into your life, cultivating positive thinking, and embracing the mind-body connection, you have the power to transform your thoughts, emotions, and ultimately your well-being.

Remember, it's a journey that requires practice, consistency, and self-compassion. Start small, be patient, and celebrate every positive shift you experience. With these practical examples and a mindset of openness, you're on your way to harnessing the incredible potential within you for healing, growth, and a vibrant life.

**NOTES :**

.........................................................................................
.........................................................................................
.........................................................................................
.........................................................................................
.........................................................................................
.........................................................................................
.........................................................................................
.........................................................................................
.........................................................................................
.........................................................................................
.........................................................................................
.........................................................................................
.........................................................................................
.........................................................................................
.........................................................................................
.........................................................................................
.........................................................................................
.........................................................................................
.........................................................................................
.........................................................................................

**NOTES :**

........................................................................................................
........................................................................................................
........................................................................................................
........................................................................................................
........................................................................................................
........................................................................................................
........................................................................................................
........................................................................................................
........................................................................................................
........................................................................................................
........................................................................................................
........................................................................................................
........................................................................................................
........................................................................................................
........................................................................................................
........................................................................................................
........................................................................................................
........................................................................................................
........................................................................................................
........................................................................................................

# *Chapter 16*

## *Understanding the Role of Exercise in Blood Sugar Management*

*This chapter will unveil the incredible benefits of exercise for blood sugar management.*

*In this fun, practical, and motivating chapter, we'll explore the role of exercise in managing blood sugar levels and share easy-to-implement daily exercises, even for the busiest of schedules.*

*Get ready to discover how exercise can be enjoyable, practical, and seamlessly integrated into your daily routine!*

## THE IMPORTANCE OF EXERCISE

Exercise plays a vital role in blood sugar management by improving insulin sensitivity, promoting weight management, reducing stress, and enhancing overall well-being. Regular physical activity can help regulate blood sugar levels, improve cardiovascular health, and increase energy levels. It's time to embrace the transformative power of exercise!

### Finding Time for Exercise

Even with a busy schedule, you can make time for exercise by adopting practical strategies:

### Incorporate Active Time Outs

Take short time outs throughout the day to engage in brief exercises. For example, take a brisk walk during your lunch time, do a few minutes of stretching or bodyweight exercises, or take the stairs instead of the elevator.

Morning Routine

Start your day with a quick workout routine. Dedicate 10-15 minutes to exercises that get your heart rate up, such as jumping jacks, jogging in place, or a quick bodyweight circuit. This jump-starts your metabolism and sets a positive tone for the day.

Utilise Commute Time

If possible, incorporate physical activity into your commute. Walk or bike to work or park your car farther away from your destination to allow for a short walk.

Break It Down

If you struggle to find large blocks of time, break your exercise sessions into shorter bursts throughout the day. Aim for three 10-minute sessions instead of one 30-minute session. These smaller bouts of activity can be just as effective.

## FUN AND PRACTICAL EXERCISES

Make exercise enjoyable and practical by incorporating activities you genuinely enjoy.

Here are some easy-to-implement exercises that can be integrated into your daily routine:

Dancing

Put on your favourite tunes and dance like nobody's watching! Dancing is a joyful and effective way to get moving and elevate your heart rate. Clear some space in your living room and have a dance party to boost your mood and burn calories.

Bodyweight Exercises

Engage in simple bodyweight exercises that require minimal equipment, such as squats, lunges, push-ups, and planks. These exercises can be done in the comfort of your home, and you can adjust the intensity to match your fitness level.

Interval Training

Incorporate short bursts of high-intensity exercises into your routine. For example, alternate between one minute of intense jumping jacks or burpees with one minute of rest or lower-intensity exercises.

This type of training can boost your metabolism and improve cardiovascular fitness.

Walking

One of the simplest and most accessible exercises, walking offers numerous health benefits.

Take brisk walks around your neighbourhood, explore local parks, or incorporate walking meetings into your work routine.

## WALKING FITNESS BEGINNER TIPS

Start Gradually

- Begin with shorter walks at a comfortable pace.
- Gradually increase your distance and speed over time.
- This will help prevent injury and allow your body to adjust to the activity

Wear Comfortable Shoes

- Proper footwear will enhance your walking experience.
- It will reduce the risk of discomfort or foot-related issues.

Warm Up and Cool Down

- Before starting your walk, spend a few minutes doing some light warm up exercises, such as stretching or marching in place.
- This will prepare your muscles for activity and reduce the chance of injury

Pay Attention to Posture

- Maintain good posture while walking.
- Good posture optimises your stride and minimises strain on your body.

Track Your Progress and Set Goals

- Monitoring your progress can be motivating and help you set realistic goals.
- Aim to gradually increase your walking duration or distance over time.
- Challenge yourself whilst still being mindful of your capabilities.

## STAY MOTIVATED AND MAKE IT FUN

To stay motivated and make exercise fun, consider the following tips:

Set Realistic Goals:

Start with small, achievable goals and gradually increase the intensity and duration of your workouts as you progress. Celebrate milestones along the way to keep yourself motivated.

Find a Workout Buddy:

Exercise with a friend or family member to make it more enjoyable and hold each other accountable. Having a workout buddy can provide support, encouragement, and make the experience more enjoyable.

Explore Variety:

Keep things interesting by trying different exercises and activities. Explore classes, online workouts, or outdoor activities that pique your interest. From swimming to hiking and cycling, there are numerous options to keep your exercise routine exciting.

Track Your Progress:
Keep a record of your exercise sessions, noting the duration, intensity, and how you felt afterward. Seeing your progress over time can be incredibly motivating and provide a sense of accomplishment.

**SUMMARY**

Congratulations on discovering the role of exercise in blood sugar management! By finding time for exercise, incorporating practical and enjoyable activities, and staying motivated, you're taking proactive steps toward managing your blood sugar levels and improving your overall health. Remember to make exercise a fun and integral part of your daily routine, embracing the variety and flexibility it offers.

With these easy-to-implement exercises and a positive mindset, you can experience the benefits of regular physical activity while having fun along the way. So, lace up your sneakers, turn up the music, and embark on a journey of vibrant health and well-being through the power of exercise!

**NOTES :**

**NOTES :**

........................................................................................................................

........................................................................................................................

........................................................................................................................

........................................................................................................................

........................................................................................................................

........................................................................................................................

........................................................................................................................

........................................................................................................................

........................................................................................................................

........................................................................................................................

........................................................................................................................

........................................................................................................................

........................................................................................................................

........................................................................................................................

........................................................................................................................

........................................................................................................................

........................................................................................................................

........................................................................................................................

........................................................................................................................

........................................................................................................................

........................................................................................................................

# *Chapter 17*

## *Designing an Exercise Routine for Diabetes Management*

*This chapter will guide you through designing an engaging exercise routine for diabetes management.*

*In this chapter, we'll provide simple steps to follow and implement, ensuring that your exercise routine is effective, enjoyable, and tailored to your individual needs.*

*Get ready to create a routine that will support your blood sugar management journey with excitement and engagement!*

### ASSESS YOUR CURRENT FITNESS LEVEL

Begin by assessing your current fitness level to determine your starting point. Consider factors such as your overall health, any existing medical conditions, and your exercise history. This self-evaluation will help you design a routine that is safe and appropriate for you.

### SET CLEAR AND REALISTIC GOALS

Define clear and realistic goals that align with your diabetes management needs. Whether it's improving cardiovascular fitness, increasing strength, or enhancing flexibility, having specific goals will keep you motivated and focused.

### CHOOSE ACTIVITIES YOU ENJOY

Select activities that you genuinely enjoy. When you engage in activities you find pleasurable, you're more likely to stick with them long term.

Experiment with different types of exercise, such as walking, cycling, swimming, dancing, or participating in team sports, until you find what brings you joy.

### INCORPORATE CARDIOVASCULAR EXERCISE

Cardiovascular exercise, also known as aerobic exercise, is crucial for improving heart health, increasing insulin sensitivity, and managing blood sugar levels. Aim for at least 150 minutes of moderate-intensity aerobic activity or 75 minutes of vigorous-intensity aerobic activity per week. Examples include brisk walking, cycling, or aerobic classes.

### INCLUDE STRENGTH TRAINING

Strength training helps build muscle, improves insulin sensitivity, and enhances overall body composition. Incorporate strength training exercises at least two days a week, targeting major muscle groups.

You can use resistance bands, free weights, or bodyweight exercises like squats, lunges, push-ups, and planks.

### PRIORITISE FLEXIBILITY AND BALANCE

Remember to include flexibility and balance exercises in your routine. These exercises improve joint mobility, reduce the risk of injuries, and promote overall physical well-being. Stretching enhances flexibility and balance.

### SCHEDULE REGULAR EXERCISE SESSIONS

Create a schedule that includes regular exercise sessions. Consistency is key for achieving your goals and maintaining blood sugar control.

Block out specific times in your week dedicated to exercise and treat them as non-negotiable appointments with yourself.

### GRADUALLY INCREASE INTENSITY

Start at a comfortable intensity level and gradually increase the intensity of your workouts as your fitness improves. This progression will challenge your body and help you achieve continuous improvements in your diabetes management.

### MONITOR YOUR BLOOD SUGAR LEVELS

Before, during, and after exercise, monitor your blood sugar levels to understand how your body responds. This will help you identify patterns, make necessary adjustments to your routine, and ensure your blood sugar remains within a safe range.

### STAY HYDRATED AND FUEL PROPERLY

Hydration and proper nutrition are essential for optimising your exercise routine. Drink plenty of water before, during, and after your workouts to stay hydrated.

Additionally, fuel your body with balanced meals and snacks to provide the necessary energy for your exercise sessions.

### STAY MOTIVATED AND ENGAGED

To stay motivated and engaged, consider the following strategies:

- Vary your exercises to prevent boredom.
- Set short-term milestones to celebrate your progress along the way.
- Keep a workout journal to track your achievements and reflect on how exercise positively impacts your diabetes management.
- Involve friends or family members by exercising together or joining group activities.

## SUMMARY

Well done on designing an engaging exercise routine for diabetes management! By following these simple steps, you've created a plan that is tailored to your needs, enjoyable, and effective.

Remember to assess your fitness level, set realistic goals, choose activities you love, incorporate cardiovascular and strength training exercises, prioritize flexibility and balance, and schedule regular workouts.

Stay motivated, monitor your blood sugar levels, fuel your body properly, and celebrate your achievements along the way.

With this engaging exercise routine, you're on your way to optimal blood sugar management, improved overall health, and a life filled with vitality and joy.

**NOTES :**

............................................................................

............................................................................

............................................................................

............................................................................

............................................................................

............................................................................

............................................................................

............................................................................

............................................................................

............................................................................

............................................................................

............................................................................

............................................................................

............................................................................

............................................................................

............................................................................

............................................................................

............................................................................

............................................................................

............................................................................

............................................................................

**NOTES :**

........................................................................................................

........................................................................................................

........................................................................................................

........................................................................................................

........................................................................................................

........................................................................................................

........................................................................................................

........................................................................................................

........................................................................................................

........................................................................................................

........................................................................................................

........................................................................................................

........................................................................................................

........................................................................................................

........................................................................................................

........................................................................................................

........................................................................................................

........................................................................................................

........................................................................................................

........................................................................................................

........................................................................................................

# *Chapter 18*

## *Incorporating Cardiovascular Exercises for Improved Blood Sugar Control*

*In this chapter,*
*novices will learn how to*
*incorporate cardiovascular*
*exercises for improved blood*
*sugar control.*

*We will provide examples of*
*beginner-friendly*
*cardiovascular exercises that*
*can be easily implemented.*

*Get ready to embark on a*
*journey of improved fitness,*
*better blood sugar control,*
*and*
*enhanced overall well-being!*

## WALKING

Walking is one of the simplest and most accessible cardiovascular exercises, making it perfect for beginners. It requires no special equipment and can be easily incorporated into your daily routine. Start with shorter walks and gradually increase your distance and pace over time.

Aim for a brisk walk where you can still hold a conversation but feel slightly breathless. You can walk outdoors in your neighbourhood, at a local park, or on a treadmill if you prefer an indoor option.

## CYCLING

Cycling is a low-impact cardiovascular exercise that provides an excellent workout for the legs and cardiovascular system. Whether you prefer outdoor cycling or using a stationary bike, it's a great option for beginners.

Start with shorter rides at a comfortable pace and gradually increase your duration and intensity. You can explore bike paths, ride around your neighbourhood, or join indoor cycling classes.

**SWIMMING**

Swimming is a fantastic cardiovascular exercise that is gentle on the joints. It provides a full-body workout while supporting your body weight, making it an ideal option for beginners.

If you're new to swimming, start with leisurely laps or water aerobics classes. As your fitness improves, gradually increase your intensity, and challenge yourself with different swimming strokes or water-based workouts.

**DANCING**

Dancing is a fun and engaging cardiovascular exercise that doesn't feel like a traditional workout.

You can choose from various dance styles such as Zumba, salsa, hip-hop, or even belly dancing. Join beginner-level dance classes or follow along with dance workout videos online. Dancing not only improves your cardiovascular health but also boosts your mood and coordination.

### LOW-IMPACT AEROBICS

Low-impact aerobic exercises provide a gentle yet effective way to get your heart rate up and improve blood sugar control. They minimise stress on your joints while still providing a cardiovascular challenge. Look for low-impact aerobics classes or follow along with online workout videos that cater to beginners. Exercises like low-impact aerobics, step aerobics, or cardio kickboxing can be excellent choices.

### ELLIPTICAL TRAINER

An elliptical trainer offers a low-impact, full-body cardiovascular workout that is beginner-friendly.

It mimics movements like walking, jogging, or climbing stairs, all while providing smooth, joint-friendly motion. Start with a comfortable resistance level and gradually increase your intensity as you become more comfortable. Incorporate short intervals of higher intensity to challenge yourself and improve cardiovascular fitness.

### JUMPING ROPE OR SKIPPING

Jumping rope is a simple yet effective cardiovascular exercise that can be done anywhere with a suitable surface. It improves coordination, cardiovascular endurance, and can be tailored to suit your fitness level. Start with shorter intervals and gradually increase your duration as you build stamina.

If jumping rope is too intense initially, try alternating between jumping and marching in place.

## *Chapter 17*

### STAIR CLIMBING

Stair climbing is an accessible cardiovascular exercise that can be performed using stairs in your home, office building, or a nearby park. Start by climbing a single flight of stairs and gradually increase your number of repetitions as your fitness improves.

If outdoor stairs are unavailable, you can use a stair climber machine at the gym or try step-ups on a sturdy platform.

Remember, it's essential to start at a comfortable level and gradually increase the intensity and duration of your workouts. Listen to your body and make modifications as needed.

Always consult with your healthcare provider before starting any new exercise program, especially if you have any underlying health conditions.

## SUMMARY

Congratulations on incorporating cardiovascular exercises into your routine for improved blood sugar control!

By choosing beginner-friendly exercises such as walking, cycling, swimming, dancing, low-impact aerobics, elliptical training, jumping rope, or stair climbing, you're taking proactive steps towards better fitness and managing your blood sugar levels effectively.

Remember to start at a comfortable level, gradually increase the intensity, and find activities that you enjoy.

Stay consistent, stay motivated, and enjoy the numerous benefits that cardiovascular exercise brings to your overall health and well-being!

## NOTES :

**NOTES :**

# *Chapter 19*

## *Strength Training and Diabetes:*

## *Building a Strong Foundation*

*Welcome to the chapter that will introduce you to the fun and practical world of strength training for diabetes management.*

*In this chapter, we'll explore how strength training can help you build a strong foundation for better health, blood sugar control, and overall well-being.*

*Get ready to discover the exciting benefits of strength training and learn practical ways to incorporate it into your diabetes management routine!*

## THE POWER OF STRENGTH TRAINING

Strength training, also known as resistance training or weightlifting, offers numerous benefits for individuals with diabetes. It helps build lean muscle mass, increases metabolism, improves insulin sensitivity, and supports weight management. Additionally, strength training enhances bone density, promotes better cardiovascular health, and boosts overall strength and functional fitness.

## START WITH PROPER FORM AND TECHNIQUE

Before diving into strength training, it's essential to learn and practice proper form and technique. This ensures optimal results and reduces the risk of injury. If you're new to strength training, consider working with a qualified fitness professional who can guide you through proper form and help design a program tailored to your needs.

## BODYWEIGHT EXERCISES

Bodyweight exercises are an excellent way to get started with strength training as they require no equipment and can be performed anywhere. They effectively engage multiple muscle groups and build strength using the resistance of your body. Some examples of bodyweight exercises include squats, lunges, push-ups, planks, and burpees. Begin with a few repetitions of each exercise and gradually increase as you build strength and confidence.

## RESISTANCE BANDS

Resistance bands are affordable, portable, and versatile tools for strength training. They provide resistance throughout the entire range of motion, targeting specific muscle groups. Use resistance bands for exercises like bicep curls, rows, shoulder presses, and lateral leg raises. They come in different resistance levels, allowing you to gradually progress as your strength improves.

## FREE WEIGHTS

Free weights, such as dumbbells or kettlebells, add an extra challenge to your strength training routine. They engage stabilizer muscles and offer a wide range of exercise options. Start with lighter weights and focus on proper form before gradually increasing the resistance. Exercises like dumbbell squats, overhead presses, deadlifts, and kettlebell swings can be incorporated into your routine.

## FUNCTIONAL TRAINING

Functional training involves exercises that mimic movements used in daily activities or sports. It improves overall strength, stability, and coordination. Incorporate exercises like squats, lunges, step-ups, and medicine ball throws to enhance your functional fitness.

This type of training can have a practical and direct impact on your daily life.

## CIRCUIT TRAINING

Circuit training combines strength exercises with cardiovascular intervals, offering a fun and efficient way to incorporate both into your routine. Create a circuit by alternating between strength exercises and short bursts of cardiovascular activities like jumping jacks, high knees, or skipping rope. This not only builds strength but also elevates your heart rate for added cardiovascular benefits.

## STAY CONSISTENT AND PROGRESS GRADUALLY

Consistency is key when it comes to strength training. Aim for at least two to three sessions per week, allowing for rest days in between. Start with lighter weights or lower resistance and gradually increase as you get stronger.

Challenge yourself without compromising proper form and always listen to your body's signals.

## TRACK YOUR PROGRESS AND CELEBRATE ACHIEVEMENTS

Keep a record of your strength training sessions, noting the exercises, weights used, and repetitions performed. Tracking your progress allows you to see how far you've come and provides motivation to continue. Celebrate your achievements along the way, whether it's lifting heavier weights, performing more repetitions, or noticing improvements in your overall strength and well-being.

## ENJOY THE JOURNEY

Above all, make strength training enjoyable and part of your lifestyle. Find exercises you enjoy and mix up your routine to keep it fun and engaging. Invite a friend or join a group class to add a social element to your strength training sessions.

Remember, the journey of building a strong foundation is as important as the results you achieve.

## SUMMARY

Congratulations on exploring the fun and practical world of strength training for diabetes management!

By incorporating bodyweight exercises, resistance bands, free weights, functional training, and circuit training, you're building a strong foundation for better health, blood sugar control, and overall well-being.

Stay consistent, focus on proper form, progress gradually, and celebrate your achievements along the way.

Enjoy the journey of strength training and embrace the positive impact it can have on your diabetes management and overall quality of life!

**NOTES :**

**NOTES :**

..........................................................................................

..........................................................................................

..........................................................................................

..........................................................................................

..........................................................................................

..........................................................................................

..........................................................................................

..........................................................................................

..........................................................................................

..........................................................................................

..........................................................................................

..........................................................................................

..........................................................................................

..........................................................................................

..........................................................................................

..........................................................................................

..........................................................................................

..........................................................................................

..........................................................................................

..........................................................................................

..........................................................................................

# *Chapter 20*

## *Flexibility and Balance Exercises for Diabetes Management*

*This chapter will introduce you to the importance of flexibility and balance exercises for diabetes management.*

*In this practical chapter, we'll explore examples of exercises that enhance flexibility and improve balance.*

*Get ready to incorporate these exercises into your routine and reap the benefits of improved mobility, stability, and overall well-being!*

## THE SIGNIFICANCE OF FLEXIBILITY AND BALANCE

Flexibility exercises help improve the range of motion in your joints, enhance muscle elasticity, and reduce the risk of injuries. Balance exercises, on the other hand, enhance stability and coordination, reducing the risk of falls and improving functional movement. Both flexibility and balance are crucial components of overall fitness and can greatly contribute to your diabetes management journey.

### STRETCHING

Stretching is a fundamental flexibility exercise that can be easily incorporated into your daily routine.

Here are a few examples of stretches to target different muscle groups:

Standing Calf Stretch: Stand near a wall, place one foot behind you, and press your heel to the ground while keeping your back leg straight.

Feel the stretch in your calf muscle. Hold for 20-30 seconds and switch sides.

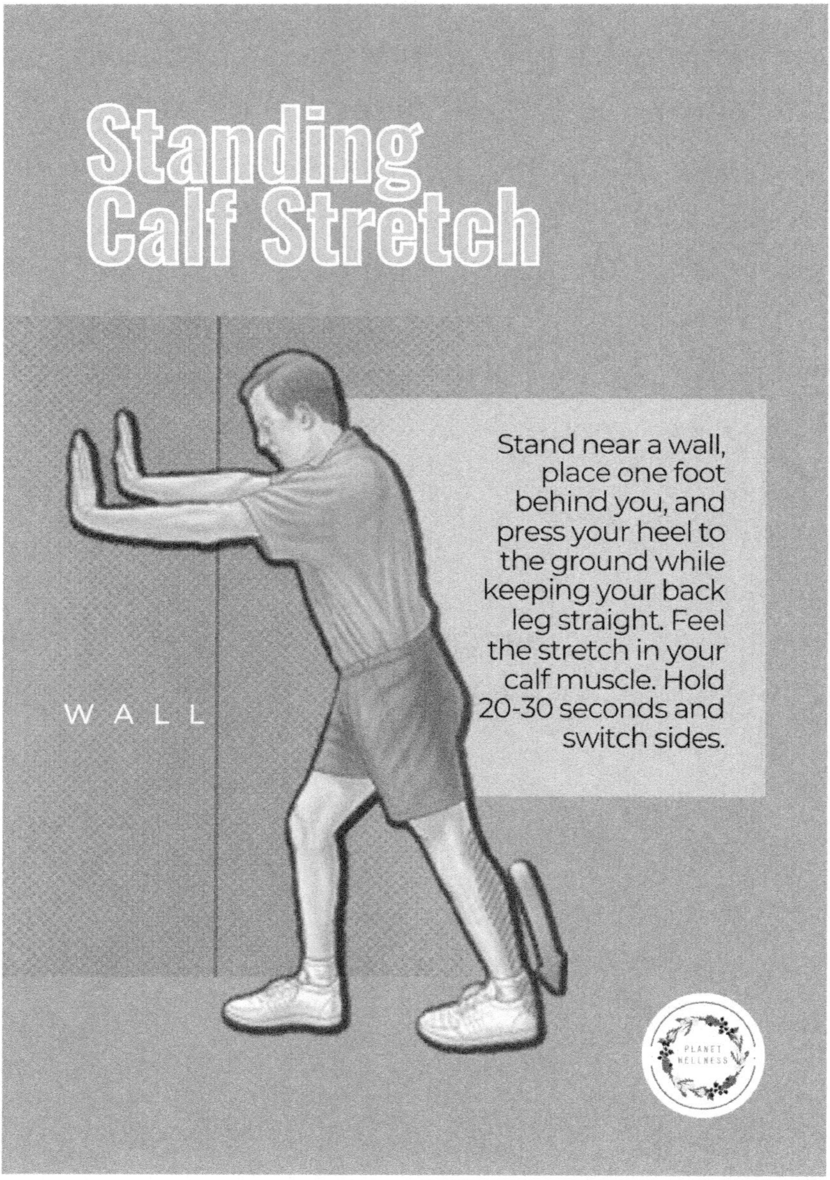

# Standing Hamstring Stretch:

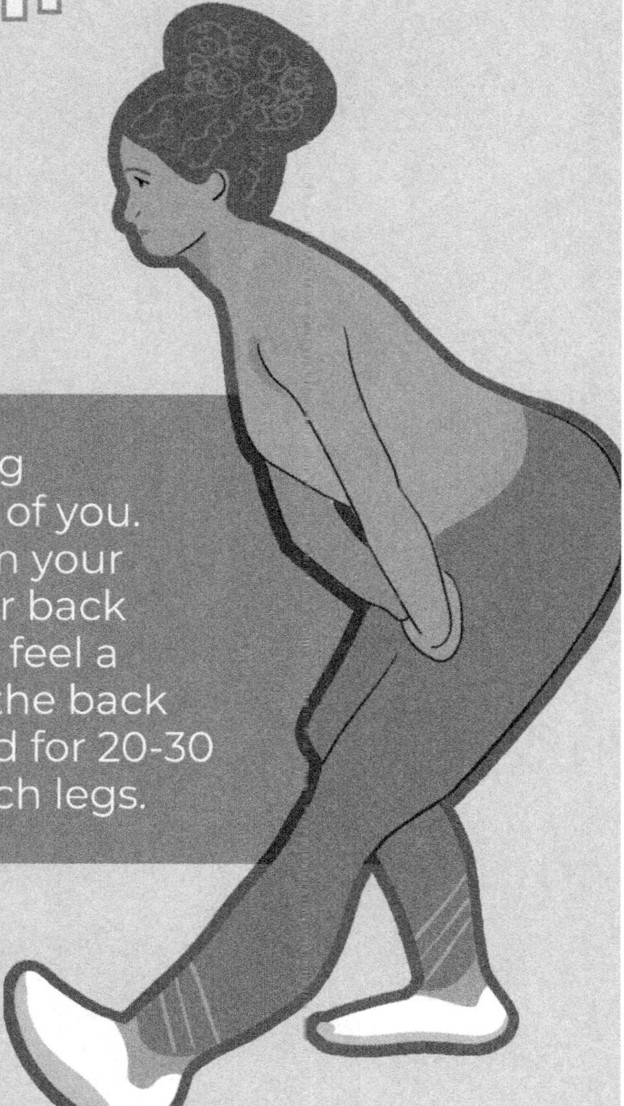

Stand with one leg extended in front of you. Lean forward from your hips, keeping your back straight, until you feel a gentle stretch in the back of your thigh. Hold for 20-30 seconds and switch legs.

# Shoulder and Chest Stretch:

Stand tall, clasp your hands behind your back, gently lift your arms away from your body while squeezing your should blades together. Feel the stretch across your chest and shoulders. Hold for 20-30 seconds.

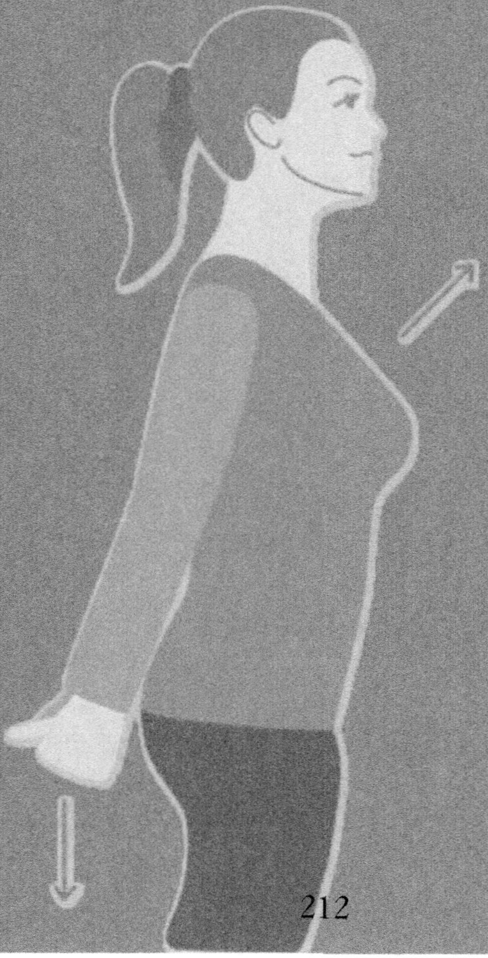

Remember to breathe deeply and relax into each stretch.

Avoid bouncing or jerking movements, and work within your range of comfort without causing pain.

# Heel-to-Toe Walk

The heel-to-toe walk is a simple yet effective exercise for improving balance and coordination. find a clear path and take steps by placing your heel directly in front of your toes with each step. Keep your gaze forward and arms relaxed by your sides. Take 10-15 steps in one direction and then reverse. For an added challenge, try walking along a straight line or a balance beam if available.

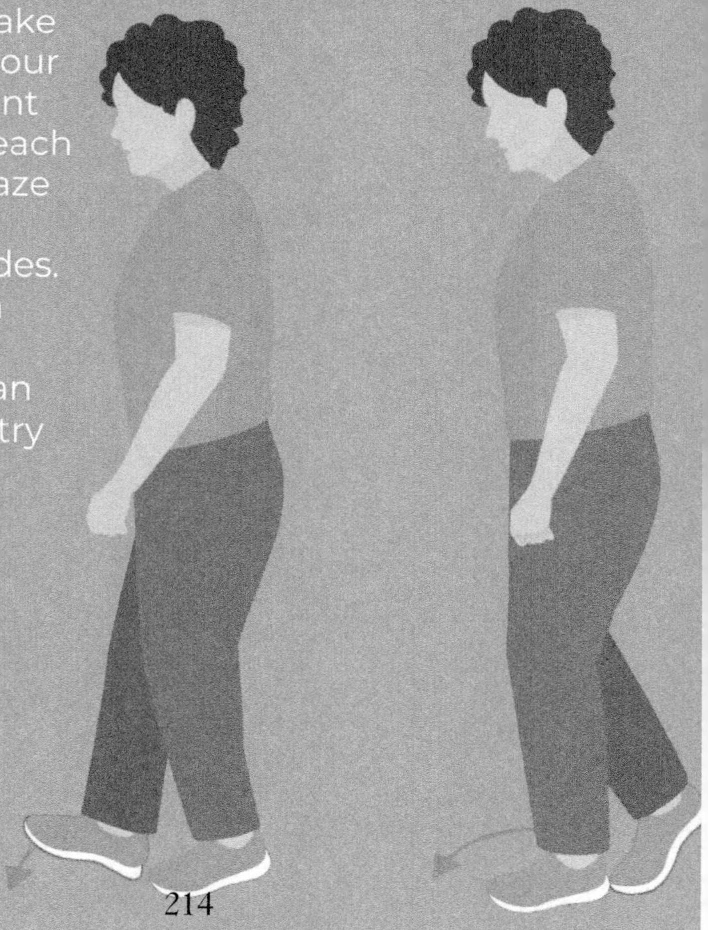

# Single-Leg Stance:

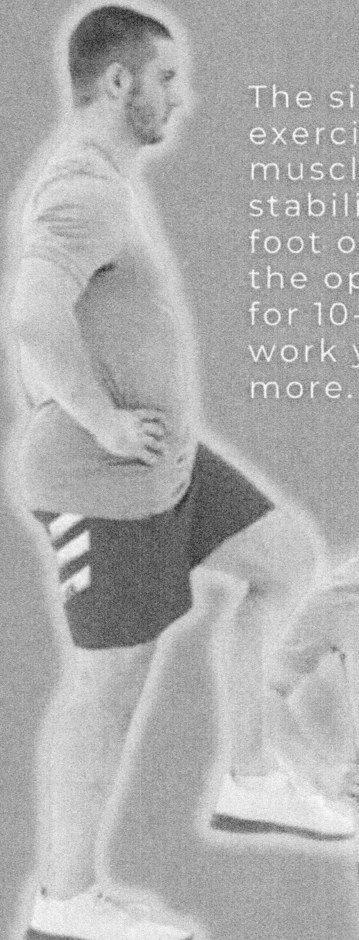

The single-leg stance is a balance exercise that helps strengthen the muscles involved in maintaining stability. Stand tall and lift one foot off the ground, balancing on the opposite leg. Start by holding for 10-15 seconds and gradually work your way up to 30 seconds or more.

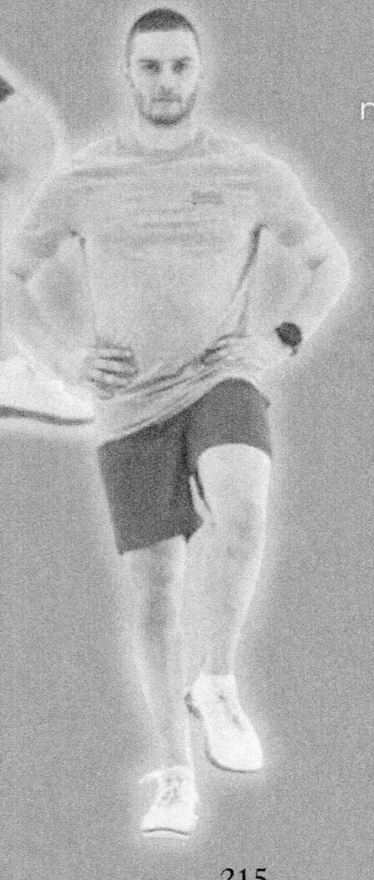

Use a wall or chair for support if needed. Switch legs and repeat. As you progress, try performing the exercise with your eyes closed to further challenge your balance.

PLANET WELLNESS

Remember to always prioritise safety and listen to your body.

Start with exercises that match your current fitness level and gradually progress as you become more comfortable.

If you have any pre-existing medical conditions or concerns, consult with your healthcare provider before beginning a new exercise routine.

## SUMMARY

Congratulations on exploring the world of flexibility and balance exercises for diabetes management! By incorporating stretching and specific balance exercises, you're enhancing your mobility, stability, and overall well-being.

Make these exercises practical by incorporating them into your daily routine, starting with beginner-friendly variations, and gradually progressing at your own pace.

Enjoy the benefits of improved flexibility, better balance, and increased confidence in your movements.

Embrace the journey of enhancing your physical abilities while managing your diabetes with grace and resilience!

**NOTES :**

# *Chapter 21*

## *Mind-Body Practices for Stress Reduction & Blood Sugar Regulation*

*This chapter will introduce you to the power of mind-body practices for stress reduction and blood sugar regulation.*

*In this easy-to-read and enjoyable chapter, we'll explore the dangers of unmanaged stress and provide examples of stress reduction practices.*

*Get ready to discover effective techniques to calm your mind, reduce stress, and support healthy blood sugar levels.*

## THE DANGERS OF UNMANAGED STRESS

Unmanaged stress can have a significant impact on your overall health, including blood sugar regulation. When you're under stress, your body releases stress hormones like cortisol and adrenaline, which can increase blood sugar levels.

Prolonged exposure to these hormones can disrupt insulin production and utilisation, leading to imbalances in blood sugar control. Additionally, chronic stress can contribute to unhealthy coping mechanisms like emotional eating, which can further disrupt blood sugar levels and contribute to weight gain.

## DEEP BREATHING

Deep breathing exercises are a simple and effective way to activate the body's relaxation response, calm the mind, and reduce stress.

Practice diaphragmatic breathing by placing one hand on your abdomen and inhaling deeply through your nose, allowing your belly to rise. Exhale slowly through your mouth, feeling your belly lower. Repeat this deep breathing pattern for several minutes, focusing on the sensation of each breath and allowing tension to melt away.

### PROGRESSIVE MUSCLE RELAXATION

Progressive muscle relaxation is a technique that involves systematically tensing and releasing different muscle groups to promote deep relaxation. Start by tensing a specific muscle group, such as your fists or shoulders, for a few seconds, and then release the tension while focusing on the sensation of relaxation.

Gradually work your way through different muscle groups, from head to toe, experiencing the release of tension and cultivating a sense of calmness.

## MINDFUL WALKING

Engage in mindful walking to reduce stress and connect with the present moment. Find a quiet and peaceful outdoor space, and as you walk, focus your attention on the sensations of each step—the feeling of your feet connecting with the ground, the rhythm of your breath, and the sights and sounds around you. Allow your mind to let go of worries and distractions, immersing yourself fully in the experience of walking.

## CREATIVE EXPRESSION

Engaging in creative activities can be an effective outlet for stress reduction. Find a creative outlet that resonates with you, such as painting, drawing, writing, playing a musical instrument, or engaging in crafts. The process of creative expression can help shift your focus away from stressors, allowing you to channel your emotions and find joy and relaxation in the present moment.

### JOURNALING

Journaling is a powerful tool for self-reflection, stress reduction, and emotional well-being. Take a few minutes each day to write down your thoughts, feelings, and experiences. Use this time to express gratitude, explore your emotions, and gain clarity on any stressors or challenges you may be facing. Journaling can provide a sense of release, promote self-awareness, and serve as a means of processing stress in a healthy way.

### ENGAGING IN HOBBIES AND LEISURE ACTIVITIES

Participating in hobbies and leisure activities that bring you joy, and relaxation is an effective way to reduce stress and support blood sugar regulation. Find activities that you genuinely enjoy, such as gardening, cooking, listening to music, reading, or engaging in sports. Dedicate regular time to these activities, allowing yourself to fully immerse in the present moment and disconnect from stressors.

Remember that finding what works for you is key. Experiment with different practices and techniques to discover which ones resonate with you the most. Incorporate these stress reduction practices into your daily routine to support healthy blood sugar regulation and promote overall well-being.

## SUMMARY

Congratulations on exploring mind-body practices for stress reduction and blood sugar regulation! By recognizing the dangers of unmanaged stress and implementing techniques like deep breathing, progressive muscle relaxation, mindful walking, creative expression, journaling, and engaging in hobbies, you're taking proactive steps to improve your well-being and support healthy blood sugar control. Embrace these enjoyable practices and let them become an integral part of your daily life. Cultivate moments of calmness, relaxation, and self-care, empowering yourself to manage stress effectively while promoting optimal blood sugar regulation and overall vitality.

**NOTES :**

# *Chapter 22*

## *Sleep and Diabetes: The Importance of Quality Rest*

*This chapter highlights the significance of quality rest in managing diabetes.*

*We explore the different levels of rest, the role of sleep in our body's repair process, and provide encouragement for the reader to prioritise and attain quality rest daily.*

*We'll also suggest natural remedies to support a good night's sleep.*

*Get ready to unlock the power of sleep for improved diabetes management and overall well-being.*

## UNDERSTANDING DIFFERENT LEVELS OF REST

Restful sleep consists of various stages, each with its own unique characteristics and benefits. These stages include light sleep, deep sleep, and rapid eye movement (REM) sleep. Light sleep acts as a transition phase, preparing the body for deeper sleep. Deep sleep is crucial for physical restoration and rejuvenation, while REM sleep supports cognitive function and emotional well-being. Achieving a balanced and enough of each stage is vital for optimal rest and overall health.

## THE BODY'S REPAIR PROCESS DURING SLEEP

While we sleep, our bodies undergo a remarkable repair process that contributes to overall well-being. During deep sleep, the body experiences tissue regeneration, muscle repair, and the release of growth hormones. This stage is particularly important for individuals with diabetes, as it aids in insulin sensitivity and blood sugar regulation.

Additionally, REM sleep promotes brain function, memory consolidation, and emotional processing. By prioritizing quality rest, we provide our bodies with the opportunity to undergo these vital repair processes.

### PRIORITISING QUALITY REST

Quality rest should be a priority in diabetes management. Here are some tips to help you achieve and maintain good sleep hygiene:

### ESTABLISH A CONSISTENT SLEEP SCHEDULE

Set a regular sleep routine by going to bed and waking up at the same time each day, even on weekends. This helps regulate your body's internal clock and promotes better sleep quality.

### CREATE A RELAXING SLEEP ENVIRONMENT

Make your bedroom a tranquil sanctuary by keeping it cool, dark, and quiet.

Consider using blackout curtains, earplugs, or a white noise machine to minimise disruptions.

### LIMIT EXPOSURE TO ELECTRONICS

Avoid using electronic devices, such as smartphones and tablets, for at least an hour before bed.

The blue light emitted by these devices can interfere with your sleep cycle. Instead, engage in calming activities like reading a book or practicing relaxation techniques.

### PRACTICE RELAXATION TECHNIQUES

Incorporate relaxation techniques into your bedtime routine to signal your body that it's time to unwind.

Deep breathing exercises, gentle stretching, or taking a warm bath can help relax both your body and mind.

### MANAGE STRESS

High levels of stress can disrupt sleep. Implement stress management strategies such as journaling, engaging in hobbies, or practicing mindfulness throughout the day to promote a more peaceful mindset before bedtime.

### NATURAL REMEDIES TO SUPPORT QUALITY SLEEP

In addition to adopting good sleep hygiene practices, natural remedies can help promote better sleep. Consider incorporating the following into your bedtime routine:

### HERBAL TEAS

Chamomile, lavender, and valerian root teas are known for their calming properties and can help promote relaxation and improve sleep quality. Sip on a cup of herbal tea before bed to unwind.

## AROMATHERAPY

Essential oils like lavender, bergamot, and chamomile can create a soothing ambiance that promotes relaxation. Use a diffuser or add a few drops of essential oil to your pillowcase to enhance your sleep environment.

## NATURAL SUPPLEMENTS

Consult with your healthcare provider about natural supplements, such as melatonin or magnesium, which can support healthy sleep patterns. Ensure proper dosage and use under professional guidance.

Remember that consistency is key when implementing these natural remedies. Experiment with different approaches to find what works best for you, as individual responses to these remedies may vary.

## SUMMARY

Congratulations on recognising the importance of quality rest in managing diabetes! By understanding the different levels of rest, appreciating the body's repair process during sleep, and implementing strategies to prioritize sleep, you're empowering yourself to achieve optimal diabetes management and overall well-being.

Make quality rest a daily priority by establishing a consistent sleep schedule, creating a relaxing sleep environment, managing stress, and incorporating natural remedies to support better sleep.

Embrace the power of sleep, and allow your body to rejuvenate, repair, and thrive, leading to improved blood sugar control and a healthier, more vibrant life.

**NOTES :**

..............................................................................................................

..............................................................................................................

..............................................................................................................

..............................................................................................................

..............................................................................................................

..............................................................................................................

..............................................................................................................

..............................................................................................................

..............................................................................................................

..............................................................................................................

..............................................................................................................

..............................................................................................................

..............................................................................................................

..............................................................................................................

..............................................................................................................

..............................................................................................................

..............................................................................................................

..............................................................................................................

..............................................................................................................

..............................................................................................................

..............................................................................................................

**NOTES :**

# *Chapter 23*

## *Managing Stress for Improved Blood Sugar Control*

*This chapter delves into the realm of stress management for improved blood sugar control.*

*In this chapter, we'll define stress and explore how it affects our health, both physically and mentally.*

*We'll also provide you with five practical examples on how to manage stress effectively.*

*Get ready to discover strategies that will empower you to reduce stress and achieve better blood sugar control.*

## UNDERSTANDING STRESS AND ITS IMPACT

Stress is a natural response that our bodies have when faced with challenging or demanding situations. While acute stress can be beneficial in certain situations, chronic or unmanaged stress can have detrimental effects on our health.

Both physically and mentally, stress can disrupt various body systems, including blood sugar regulation. High levels of stress hormones like cortisol can raise blood sugar levels and contribute to insulin resistance. Moreover, stress can lead to emotional eating, poor sleep, decreased physical activity, and unhealthy coping mechanisms, all of which can further impact blood sugar control.

## PRACTICE STRESS MANAGEMENT TECHNIQUES

Managing stress is essential for achieving better blood sugar control and overall well-being.

Here are five practical examples of stress management techniques you can incorporate into your daily life:

1.Mindfulness Meditation:

Engage in mindfulness meditation to cultivate a present-moment awareness and reduce stress. Set aside a few minutes each day to sit quietly, focus on your breath, and observe your thoughts without judgment. This practice can help calm the mind, reduce anxiety, and promote a sense of inner peace.

2.Physical Activity:

Engaging in regular physical activity is a powerful stress management tool. Exercise releases endorphins, which are natural mood boosters, and helps reduce stress levels. Find activities you enjoy, such as walking, dancing, swimming, or cycling, and aim for at least 30 minutes of moderate intensity exercise most days of the week.

3.Deep Breathing Exercises:

Deep breathing exercises can activate the body's relaxation response and help reduce stress. Practice diaphragmatic breathing by inhaling deeply through your nose, allowing your belly to rise, and exhaling slowly through your mouth.

This technique promotes relaxation, lowers heart rate, and calms the nervous system.

4.Social Support:

Seek support from family, friends, or support groups to alleviate stress. Talking to someone who understands and empathizes with your situation can provide comfort and perspective.

Engage in activities that promote social connections, such as sharing a meal, participating in group activities, or joining support networks.

5.Time Management:

Effective time management can help reduce stress by allowing you to prioritise tasks, avoid overwhelm, and create a sense of control. Break tasks into smaller, manageable steps, delegate when possible, and set realistic deadlines.

Prioritise self-care activities and ensure you have time for rest and relaxation.

6.Prioritise Self-Care:

Self-care plays a crucial role in stress management. Take care of yourself physically, emotionally, and mentally to reduce stress levels.

This may include getting enough sleep, eating balanced meals, engaging in activities you enjoy, setting boundaries, practicing relaxation techniques, and scheduling regular breaks to recharge.

7.Seek Professional Help:

If stress becomes overwhelming or begins to significantly impact your daily life, consider seeking professional help. Therapists, counsellors, or healthcare providers can provide guidance and support tailored to your specific needs. They can help you develop effective coping strategies and offer valuable insights into managing stress and blood sugar control.

To have a short chat with us, do book in via https://calendly.com/wellnessiridology

**ENGAGE IN STRESS-REDUCING ACTIVITIES**

Find activities that help you relax and reduce stress. These can include hobbies, reading, listening to music, taking a bath, spending time in nature, engaging in creative pursuits, or simply dedicating time to do something you love.These activities provide an outlet for stress, promote relaxation, and contribute to overall well-being.

## SUMMARY

By understanding the impact of stress on blood sugar control and implementing effective stress management techniques, you're taking proactive steps toward achieving better overall health and improved diabetes management. Define stress, recognise its physical and mental effects, and prioritise stress reduction strategies in your daily life.

Practice
·Mindfulness,
·Engage in physical activity,
·Incorporate deep breathing exercises,
·Seek social support,
·Manage your time effectively,
·Prioritise self-care and
·Peek professional help when needed.

Remember, managing stress is a journey, so be patient and kind to yourself as you embrace these stress management techniques for enhanced blood sugar control and a happier, healthier life.

**NOTES :**

**NOTES :**

# *Chapter 24*

## *Blood Sugar Monitoring & Medication Management*

*This chapter emphasises the importance of monitoring blood sugar levels and managing medication for effective diabetes management.*

*We discuss the significance of blood sugar monitoring, define acceptable non-diabetic and pre-diabetic readings, explore different types of medication, and shed light on the potential risks of relying solely on chemical medications.*

*We will highlight how following natural solutions can empower individuals to gradually reduce their reliance on harmful drugs and achieve better long-term health outcomes.*

## IMPORTANCE OF BLOOD SUGAR MONITORING

Regular blood sugar monitoring is a fundamental aspect of diabetes management. It allows individuals to track their blood sugar levels, assess the effectiveness of their lifestyle interventions, and make necessary adjustments to maintain optimal blood sugar control.

Monitoring helps identify patterns, understand the impact of meal choices, physical activity, and stress on blood sugar levels, and empowers individuals to take proactive steps towards achieving their blood sugar goals.

## ACCEPTABLE NON-DIABETIC AND PRE-DIABETIC READINGS

For individuals without diabetes, the acceptable range for fasting blood sugar levels typically falls between 70 to 99 mg/dL (3.9 to 5.5 mmol/L).

Pre-diabetes refers to a condition where blood sugar levels are higher than normal but not yet in the diabetic range.

Pre-diabetic readings often range from 100 to 125 mg/dL (5.6 to 6.9 mmol/L) for fasting blood sugar levels. It's essential to monitor blood sugar levels regularly and consult with healthcare professionals to determine individualised target ranges.

## TYPES OF MEDICATION

In diabetes management, medication can play a crucial role in achieving blood sugar control. Common types of medication include:

Oral Medications:

These medications, such as metformin, sulfonylureas, and DPP-4 inhibitors, help lower blood sugar levels by increasing insulin production, improving insulin sensitivity, or reducing glucose production in the liver.

Injectable Medications:

Injectable medications like glucagon-like peptide-1 receptor agonists (GLP-1 agonists) or sodium-glucose cotransporter-2 inhibitors (SGLT-2 inhibitors) are often prescribed to assist with blood sugar control by increasing insulin secretion, reducing glucose absorption, or promoting weight loss.

Insulin Therapy:

For individuals with type 1 diabetes or those with type 2 diabetes who cannot achieve optimal blood sugar control with oral or injectable medications alone, insulin therapy may be necessary. Insulin helps regulate blood sugar levels by facilitating glucose uptake into cells.

Rethinking Medication Reliance:

While medication can be beneficial, it's essential to recognise the potential risks of relying solely on chemical medications.

Long-term reliance on these drugs may come with side effects and can sometimes lead to a sense of dependency. However, it's important to note that medication decisions should be made in consultation with healthcare professionals who have a comprehensive understanding of individual health circumstances.

## THE ROLE OF NATURAL SOLUTIONS

Embracing natural solutions, such as lifestyle modifications and holistic approaches, can be a powerful complement to medication management. By following a balanced and nutritious meal plan, engaging in regular physical activity, managing stress levels, obtaining quality rest, and incorporating other natural strategies discussed in this book, individuals can improve blood sugar control and potentially reduce their reliance on harmful drugs over time.

It's crucial to consult with healthcare professionals to ensure a safe and gradual transition.

## SUMMARY

Monitoring blood sugar levels and managing medication are essential components of diabetes management. Regular blood suga· monitoring provides valuable insights into blood sugar control patterns, enabling individuals to make informed decisions about their lifestyle and medication management.

While medication can be a helpful tool, it's important to recognise the potential risks associated with long-term reliance on chemical medications. By embracing natural solutions, individuals can empower themselves to make positive lifestyle changes, reduce medication reliance over time, and achieve better long-term health outcomes.

Remember to consult with healthcare professionals to develop a personalised plan that incorporates natural solutions while ensuring effective blood sugar control.

**NOTES :**

.................................................................................................
.................................................................................................
.................................................................................................
.................................................................................................
.................................................................................................
.................................................................................................
.................................................................................................
.................................................................................................
.................................................................................................
.................................................................................................
.................................................................................................
.................................................................................................
.................................................................................................
.................................................................................................
.................................................................................................
.................................................................................................
.................................................................................................
.................................................................................................
.................................................................................................
.................................................................................................
.................................................................................................

# *Chapter 25*

## *Support Systems & Resources for Diabetes Care*

*This chapter highlights the importance of support systems and resources for diabetes care.*

*In this chapter, we'll explore the valuable role that support networks, educational resources, and professional assistance play in effectively managing diabetes.*

*Discover the power of a strong support system and the wealth of resources available to help you navigate your diabetes journey with confidence and knowledge.*

# *Chapter 25*

Healthcare Providers:

Your healthcare team, including doctors, nurses, and diabetes educators, can provide invaluable guidance and support. Regular appointments allow you to discuss concerns, ask questions, and receive personalised advice.

Educational Resources:

Knowledge is empowering in diabetes care. Educate yourself about the condition, treatment options, lifestyle modifications, and self-care practices.

Here are some educational resources to consider:

Books and Publications:

Explore books, magazines, and websites dedicated to diabetes care and management. Look for reputable sources that provide evidence-based information and practical tips.

Online Communities and Websites:

Join online diabetes communities and visit trusted websites that offer reliable information, forums, blogs, and educational resources. Examples include the American Diabetes Association (ADA), the International Diabetes Federation (IDF), and Diabetes Self-Management.

Diabetes Education Programs:

Participate in structured diabetes education programs offered by healthcare facilities or community organisations. These programs provide comprehensive information, self-management strategies, and guidance on various aspects of diabetes care.

## PROFESSIONAL ASSISTANCE

In addition to your primary healthcare provider, consider seeking specialised professional assistance to optimise your diabetes care.

Nutritionists

Consult with a nutritionist who specializes in diabetes care. They can help develop personalised meal plans, provide nutritional guidance, and support healthy eating habits.

Diabetes Educators

Diabetes educators are trained professionals who can provide comprehensive education and guidance on managing diabetes. They can assist with medication management, blood sugar monitoring, lifestyle modifications, and problem-solving.

Mental Health Professionals

Diabetes can sometimes impact mental well-being. Seek support from mental health professionals, such as therapists or counsellors, who can help address the emotional and psychological aspects of living with diabetes.

## MOBILE APPLICATIONS AND TECHNOLOGICAL TOOLS

Leverage technology to enhance your diabetes care. Mobile applications and digital tools can assist with blood sugar tracking, medication reminders, meal planning, and even connecting with support networks. Explore reputable apps and tools that align with your specific needs and preferences.

## SUMMARY

Managing diabetes requires support, knowledge, and access to resources that empower you to take control of your health. Build a support system of family, friends, and diabetes support groups who understand and motivate you. Educate yourself through books, online communities, and educational programs to enhance your knowledge.

Seek professional assistance from Nutritionists, diabetes educators, and mental health professionals who specialise in diabetes care.

Embrace the convenience of mobile applications and technological tools designed to streamline your diabetes management.

Remember, you are not alone in your diabetes journey, and with the right support and resources, you can confidently navigate the path to optimal diabetes care.

**NOTES :**

........................................................................................................
........................................................................................................
........................................................................................................
........................................................................................................
........................................................................................................
........................................................................................................
........................................................................................................
........................................................................................................
........................................................................................................
........................................................................................................
........................................................................................................
........................................................................................................
........................................................................................................
........................................................................................................
........................................................................................................
........................................................................................................
........................................................................................................
........................................................................................................
........................................................................................................
........................................................................................................
........................................................................................................

**NOTES :**

........................................................................................................................................
........................................................................................................................................
........................................................................................................................................
........................................................................................................................................
........................................................................................................................................
........................................................................................................................................
........................................................................................................................................
........................................................................................................................................
........................................................................................................................................
........................................................................................................................................
........................................................................................................................................
........................................................................................................................................
........................................................................................................................................
........................................................................................................................................
........................................................................................................................................
........................................................................................................................................
........................................................................................................................................
........................................................................................................................................
........................................................................................................................................
........................................................................................................................................
........................................................................................................................................

# *Chapter 26*

## *Overcoming Obstacles & Staying Motivated*

*This chapter addresses the common obstacles faced in managing diabetes and provides strategies to stay motivated and on track in preventing or reversing diabetes naturally.*

*In this chapter, we'll explore hurdles such as overwhelm, time management, and peer pressure that can compromise your health.*

*Discover effective techniques to overcome these challenges and maintain the motivation needed to achieve your diabetes management goals.*

## OVERCOMING OVERWHELM

Managing diabetes can feel overwhelming at times. However, remember that small steps lead to significant progress.

Here's how you can overcome overwhelm:

### Set Realistic Goals

Break down your goals into manageable steps. Prioritise and focus on one goal at a time, whether it's adopting a healthier eating plan, increasing physical activity, or improving stress management.

### Seek Support

Lean on your support system, healthcare providers, or diabetes educators for guidance and assistance. They can help you navigate challenges, answer questions, and provide the encouragement needed to stay on track.

Educate Yourself

Expand your knowledge about diabetes management and prevention. Understanding the condition empowers you to make informed decisions and feel more in control of your health.

Celebrate Progress

Acknowledge and celebrate your achievements, no matter how small they may seem. Rewarding yourself along the way can boost motivation and keep you moving forward.

Effective Time Management

Balancing diabetes management with other responsibilities can be challenging. Here are some strategies for effective time management:

Prioritise Self-Care

Make self-care a priority by scheduling time for exercise, meal planning, stress reduction, and restful sleep.

Treat these activities as non-negotiable commitments to your health.

Plan

Plan your meals, snacks, and physical activity in advance. Use meal prepping techniques to save time during busy periods, and schedule physical activity sessions in your calendar to ensure they are not overlooked.

Delegate and Ask for Help

If possible, delegate tasks or ask for assistance from family members or friends. This can free up time and reduce the feeling of being overwhelmed.

Use Technology and Tools

Leverage technology to streamline your diabetes management. Use smartphone apps for meal tracking, blood sugar monitoring, and medication reminders. Explore tools that simplify meal planning and help manage your schedule efficiently.

## NAVIGATING PEER PRESSURE AND ENJOYING LIFE

Social situations and peer pressure can sometimes make it challenging to maintain a healthy lifestyle.

Here's how to navigate such situations while staying true to your goals:

Communicate Your Needs: Clearly communicate your dietary restrictions and health goals to friends, family, and colleagues. Help them understand your commitment to managing diabetes and ask for their support.

Plan Ahead: When attending social events or eating out, plan ahead by reviewing menus and choosing healthier options in advance. If necessary, eat a small snack before the event to avoid making impulsive, unhealthy choices.

Seek Healthy Alternatives: Look for healthier alternatives to popular indulgent foods and drinks.

Experiment with recipes that offer healthier versions of your favourite dishes or opt for lower-sugar beverages when socialising.

Find Supportive Networks: Connect with individuals who share similar health goals and can provide support during challenging times. Join diabetes support groups or online communities where you can find understanding, encouragement, and advice.

Staying Motivated: Maintaining motivation is essential for long-term success in diabetes management. Consider the following strategies to stay motivated:

Set Meaningful Goals: Define your goals in a way that aligns with your values and personal motivations. Remind yourself of the positive impact that achieving these goals will have on your health and quality of life.

Track Your Progress: Keep a record of your successes, no matter how small.

Track your blood sugar readings, physical activity achievements, and healthy food choices. Seeing your progress can reinforce your motivation.

Find Inspiration: Surround yourself with sources of inspiration. Read success stories, watch motivational videos, or listen to podcasts related to diabetes management. Connecting with others who have achieved success can ignite your motivation.

Practice Self-Care: Take care of your physical, emotional, and mental well-being. Engage in activities that bring you joy, practice relaxation techniques, and prioritize stress management. A well-nurtured self is more likely to stay motivated.

Celebrate Milestones: Celebrate milestones and achievements along your journey. Treat yourself to non-food rewards, such as a massage, a new workout outfit, or a day spent doing activities you love.

## SUMMARY

Overcoming obstacles and staying motivated in diabetes management is a continuous process that requires commitment and resilience.

By breaking tasks into manageable steps, seeking support, effectively managing your time, navigating peer pressure, and staying motivated, you can prevent or reverse diabetes naturally.

Remember, small changes add up to significant improvements in your health.

Stay focused, celebrate your successes, and enjoy the journey towards optimal health and well-being.

**NOTES :**

........................................................................................

........................................................................................

........................................................................................

........................................................................................

........................................................................................

........................................................................................

........................................................................................

........................................................................................

........................................................................................

........................................................................................

........................................................................................

........................................................................................

........................................................................................

........................................................................................

........................................................................................

........................................................................................

........................................................................................

........................................................................................

........................................................................................

........................................................................................

........................................................................................

# *Chapter 27*

## *Celebrating Success & Long-Term Lifestyle Changes*

*Welcome to the chapter that emphasises the importance of celebrating success and offers tips for maintaining and managing long-term lifestyle changes.*

*In this enjoyable chapter, we'll explore eight creative ways to celebrate your achievements and provide eight practical tips to ensure that your positive lifestyle changes become lasting habits.*

*Get ready to celebrate your progress and embrace a healthier, happier future.*

## PART 1: CELEBRATING SUCCESS

Share Your Achievements:

Share your successes with your support system, whether it's family, friends, or a diabetes support group. Let them celebrate your accomplishments and acknowledge the effort you've put into making positive changes.

Treat Yourself:

Reward yourself with non-food rewards that align with your health goals. Consider treating yourself to a spa day, a new book, a massage, a concert, or a day spent engaging in your favourite hobby.

Create a Milestone Jar:

Start a milestone jar and fill it with small notes detailing your achievements. Whenever you reach a milestone or make progress, add a note to the jar.

Whenever you need a boost of motivation, revisit your jar, and reflect on how far you've come.

Document Your Journey:

Keep a visual record of your progress, such as before-and-after photos, measurements, or journal entries. Seeing the transformation over time can be incredibly motivating and provide a sense of pride and accomplishment.

Plan a Healthy Get-Together:

Celebrate your success by organising a healthy gathering with your loved ones. Prepare nutritious meals, try out new healthy recipes, and engage in activities that promote well-being, such as group walks, dancing, or outdoor games.

Treat Yourself to a Healthy Splurge:

Indulge in a special, healthy treat. It could be a delicious fruit platter, a homemade smoothie, or a healthy version of your favourite dessert.

Savour the flavours and celebrate your dedication to making healthier choices.

Create a Vision Board:

Make a vision board that represents your long-term health and wellness goals. Use images, quotes, and affirmations to visually depict the life you aspire to. Place it somewhere visible as a daily reminder of your journey and accomplishments.

Reflect and Express Gratitude:

Take time to reflect on your progress and express gratitude for your achievements. Write down a list of things you're grateful for, including the positive changes you've made in your life. Cultivating gratitude can enhance your sense of well-being and motivation.

## PART 2: MAINTAINING LONG-TERM LIFESTYLE CHANGES

Set Realistic and Sustainable Goals:

Ensure your goals are realistic and attainable, considering your lifestyle, preferences, and capabilities. Setting achievable goals will boost your confidence and motivation to maintain long-term changes.

Build a Supportive Environment:

Surround yourself with a supportive environment that aligns with your goals. Choose friends and family members who encourage and support your healthy lifestyle choices. Engage in activities and join communities that foster a positive and health-conscious mindset.

Establish Healthy Habits:

Focus on building healthy habits that become second nature over time. Consistency is key.

Incorporate regular physical activity, mindful eating, stress management techniques, and adequate rest into your daily routine.

Keep Learning and Stay Updated:

Stay informed about the latest research, developments, and strategies related to diabetes management. Continuously educate yourself about healthy eating, exercise, stress reduction, and self-care. Attend seminars, workshops, or webinars to expand your knowledge.

Find Joy in the Journey:

Embrace the process and find joy in the small victories along the way. Shift your mindset from focusing solely on the end result to appreciating the daily progress and positive changes you're making.

Celebrate each step of your journey.

Practice Mindful Eating:

Cultivate a mindful eating practice that promotes awareness of your body's hunger and fullness cues. Pay attention to the flavours, textures, and nourishment of the foods you consume. Eat with intention and savour each bite.

Stay Active and Engaged:

Incorporate physical activity into your daily routine and make it enjoyable. Find activities you love, whether it's dancing, swimming, hiking, or playing a sport. Engage in regular movement that brings you pleasure and supports your overall well-being.

Regularly Evaluate and Adjust:

Periodically evaluate your progress and adjust your approach as needed. Assess what's working well and what may need improvement. Embrace flexibility and adapt your strategies to maintain long-term success.

## SUMMARY

Celebrating success and maintaining long-term lifestyle changes are essential elements of a fulfilling diabetes management journey.

Embrace various ways to celebrate your achievements, and make sure to find joy in the process.

Set realistic goals, build a supportive environment, establish healthy habits, and continue learning to maintain your positive lifestyle changes.

Remember, every step forward is a step toward a healthier, happier life.

Enjoy the journey, embrace the changes, and celebrate your ongoing commitment to your well-being.

**NOTES :**

# *Chapter 28*

## *The Future of Diabetes Care: Innovations and Hope*

*This chapter explores the exciting innovations and hopeful advancements in the field of diabetes care.*

*In this chapter, we'll discuss five fascinating facts about the future of diabetes care and provide you with five inspiring examples of innovations that offer hope for improved diabetes management and quality of life.*

*Get ready to envision a brighter future in diabetes care.*

# Chapter 28

## FACT: PERSONALISED MEDICINE IS ON THE RISE

In the future, advancements in technology and genetic research will allow for personalised medicine tailored to everyone's unique needs. Personalised approaches may include targeted therapies, precision nutrition, and customised treatment plans based on genetic and lifestyle factors.

## FACT: ARTIFICIAL INTELLIGENCE (AI) AND MACHINE LEARNING WILL REVOLUTIONISE DIABETES CARE

AI and machine learning hold immense potential in revolutionising diabetes care. These technologies can analyse large amounts of data, detect patterns, and provide real-time insights for personalized diabetes management.

AI-powered systems can support early detection of complications, optimise treatment plans, and enhance decision-making for healthcare providers.

## FACT: CONTINUOUS GLUCOSE MONITORING (CGM) TECHNOLOGY IS EVOLVING

Continuous Glucose Monitoring (CGM) technology is advancing rapidly, offering improved accuracy, convenience, and user-friendly features. Future innovations may include smaller, more comfortable sensors, closed-loop systems that automatically adjust insulin delivery, and integration with smartphone apps and wearable devices for seamless monitoring and data analysis.

## FACT: REGENERATIVE MEDICINE HOLDS PROMISE FOR BETA CELL RESTORATION

Regenerative medicine, a field focused on stimulating the body's natural healing processes, holds promise for restoring and regenerating pancreatic beta cells, which produce insulin. Researchers are exploring innovative approaches such as stem cell therapy, tissue engineering, and gene therapy to restore beta cell function and potentially provide a cure for diabetes.

## FACT: SMART INSULIN AND INSULIN-RELATED INNOVATIONS ARE EMERGING

Scientists and engineers are developing smart insulin formulations and delivery systems that can better mimic the body's natural insulin response. These innovations aim to improve insulin efficacy, reduce the risk of hypoglycaemia, and enhance convenience for individuals with diabetes. Examples include glucose-responsive insulin, inhalable insulin, and implantable insulin pumps.

Now, let's explore five inspiring examples of innovations and advancements in diabetes care:

### ARTIFICIAL PANCREAS SYSTEMS

Artificial pancreas systems, also known as closed-loop systems, combine continuous glucose monitoring (CGM) with insulin delivery to automate insulin dosing.

These systems can mimic the function of a healthy pancreas by adjusting insulin delivery based on real-time glucose levels, improving blood sugar control, and reducing the burden of diabetes management.

### TELEMEDICINE AND DIGITAL HEALTH SOLUTIONS

Telemedicine and digital health solutions offer convenient access to healthcare professionals, education, and support through virtual platforms. These technologies enable remote monitoring, virtual consultations, and personalised care, empowering individuals with diabetes to manage their condition from the comfort of their homes.

### GLUCOSE-RESPONSIVE INSULIN

Researchers are developing glucose-responsive insulin formulations that activate in response to high blood sugar levels and deactivate when glucose levels normalize.

This innovative insulin can provide more precise blood sugar control and reduce the risk of hypoglycaemia, enhancing the safety and effectiveness of insulin therapy.

### SMART DIABETES MANAGEMENT APPS

Smartphone apps equipped with advanced algorithms and machine learning capabilities can analyse data from CGM devices, insulin pumps, and other health trackers to provide real-time insights, personalized recommendations, and reminders. These apps empower individuals to make informed decisions, track their progress, and gain better control over their diabetes management.

### ARTIFICIAL INTELLIGENCE FOR PREDICTIVE ANALYTICS

Artificial intelligence algorithms can analyse data patterns, historical data, and lifestyle factors to predict blood sugar fluctuations and provide personalized recommendations.

These predictive analytics can assist individuals in proactively managing their diabetes, preventing potential complications, and optimising their treatment plans.

## SUMMARY

The future of diabetes care is filled with exciting innovations and hopeful advancements that promise to transform the landscape of diabetes management. From personalised medicine and AI-driven technologies to regenerative medicine and smart insulin innovations, the possibilities are vast.

Embrace the hope and optimism that these advancements bring, knowing that researchers and innovators are dedicated to improving diabetes care and enhancing the quality of life for individuals with diabetes. As we look ahead, let us anticipate a future where diabetes management becomes more precise, convenient, and ultimately leads to better health outcomes for all.

**NOTES :**

....................................................................................................

....................................................................................................

....................................................................................................

....................................................................................................

....................................................................................................

....................................................................................................

....................................................................................................

....................................................................................................

....................................................................................................

....................................................................................................

....................................................................................................

....................................................................................................

....................................................................................................

....................................................................................................

....................................................................................................

....................................................................................................

....................................................................................................

....................................................................................................

....................................................................................................

....................................................................................................

....................................................................................................

**NOTES :**

........................................................................................
........................................................................................
........................................................................................
........................................................................................
........................................................................................
........................................................................................
........................................................................................
........................................................................................
........................................................................................
........................................................................................
........................................................................................
........................................................................................
........................................................................................
........................................................................................
........................................................................................
........................................................................................
........................................................................................
........................................................................................
........................................................................................
........................................................................................
........................................................................................

# *Conclusion*

## *Overcoming Obstacles & Staying Motivated*

*CONGRATULATIONS*
*on completing the 28-day action plan for lowering blood sugar naturally!*

*As you conclude this transformative journey, it's crucial to maintain the positive changes you've implemented and sustain a healthy lifestyle in the long run.*

*In this concluding chapter, we'll provide you with eight practical action steps that you can implement to sustain a healthy lifestyle beyond the initial 28 days.*

### SET REALISTIC AND SUSTAINABLE GOALS

Continually set realistic and attainable goals that align with your health aspirations. Break them down into smaller milestones and celebrate each achievement along the way.

### MAINTAIN CONSISTENT BLOOD SUGAR MONITORING

Continue monitoring your blood sugar levels regularly, even beyond the initial 28-day plan. This practice will help you stay aware of your progress and make necessary adjustments to your lifestyle, meals, and medication as needed.

### EMBRACE VARIETY IN YOUR MEALS

Continue to prioritise a well-balanced meal that includes a variety of nutrient-rich foods. Incorporate fruits, vegetables, whole grains, lean proteins, and healthy fats into your meals to ensure you're getting a wide range of essential nutrients.

### STAY PHYSICALLY ACTIVE

Make physical activity a regular part of your routine. Aim for at least 150 minutes of moderate-intensity aerobic exercise per week, along with strength training exercises to maintain muscle mass and support overall health.

### PRACTICE MINDFUL EATING

Continue practicing mindful eating to cultivate a healthy relationship with food. Pay attention to your body's hunger and fullness cues, savour the flavours and textures of your meals, and eat with intention and gratitude.

### MANAGE STRESS EFFECTIVELY

Recognise the importance of stress management in maintaining overall health. Incorporate stress reduction techniques such as deep breathing, meditation, yoga, or engaging in activities that bring you joy and relaxation.

### FOSTER A SUPPORTIVE ENVIRONMENT

Surround yourself with a supportive network of friends, family, or fellow individuals managing diabetes. Seek encouragement and accountability from those who understand your journey and can provide ongoing support.

### REGULARLY REVIEW AND ADJUST YOUR PLAN

Periodically review your progress, reassess your goals, and adjust your action plan as needed. Life is dynamic, and your needs may change over time, so be adaptable and flexible in your approach.

Remember, sustaining a healthy lifestyle is not about perfection but about making consistent, conscious choices that support your overall well-being.

Implementing these action steps beyond the initial 28 days will help you maintain optimal blood sugar control and continue a path of improved health.

As you move forward, stay motivated, celebrate your successes, and seek inspiration from the progress you've made.

Remember that every small step contributes to significant long-term changes. Embrace the journey, stay committed to your health, and know that you have the power to sustain a healthy lifestyle beyond the 28-day action plan.

Wishing you continued success and a vibrant, diabetes-free future!

**NOTES :**

# *Bonus Section*

**FOOD FACTS TO BE AWARE OF:**

- Rice eaters can become lazy and indolent without other things in the diet. They become feeble and lose their quickness. Rice isn't a stimulating food.

- Eating red meat raises the blood pressure.

- Using fruit to a high degree can lead to nerve starvation. This is because the nerves are fed by protein. Proteins are a brain and nerve food.

- Each food has its effect on the body.

- Sulphur brings heat to the body, and heat is needed in the extremities. Always have sulphur foods with the brain foods. It will drive them to the brain.

- Dr Denis P. Burkitt linked England's increased consumption of refined carbohydrates in the 50's,60's,70's,80's,90's and to date, to increasing obesity, diabetes, diverticulitis, appendicitis and even atherosclerosis.

- In Diabetes, HCL (Hydrochloric acid) is said to bring about normal acidity to help restore natural secretion of insulin. Insulin can only function in an acid medium, so it aids the pH balance.

- Those whose health is endangered by sugar should realise that the answer is not to take another dangerous substance. We find saccharin is a coal-tar product, and all coal-tar products are carcinogenic in their activity. The big problem today is not so much in taking care of the disease, but in refusing to give up foods and activities that we know are strongly linked to disease.

- Monosodium glutamate (MSG) is an additive that has been under consideration for years as health hazard. Biochemists at Washington University found in 1969 that big doses damaged brain cells in young mice.

- As a result of these findings, some manufacturers withdrew the additive MSG from their products, especially baby foods.

- MSG is used heavily in flavour restoration for canned, packaged, frozen and precooked convenience foods. Chinese cooking uses MSG commonly. One fourth teaspoon of MSG can produce side-effects according to reports, such as allergies and digestion distress.

- 12 ounces or 340 grams of tomato juice contains Vitamin A, Ascorbic acid, Riboflavin, calcium, iron, protein, and thiamine and less calories and carbohydrates, compared to 8 ounces or 227 grams of cola drinks.

## RECOMMENDED FOODS

We also highly recommend you check out and consume the following non exhaustive list of foods at least a few times weekly.

Almond Nut Butter
A teaspoon is good to add to a drink or a small piece of goats' cheese, the size of a golf ball. Proteins of this kind are digested better in these combinations and make good tissue builders.

Beans
Kidney beans, pinto beans, black beans, and chickpeas are high in fibre and take a long time to digest. Dried beans are a better choice than canned as they are more affordable and contain less sodium.

Berries
Blueberries, raspberries, strawberries, and blackberries are packed with antioxidants, vitamins, and fibre. They can be a great healthy option to satisfy your sweet tooth.

Broccoli

This can be eaten raw and gently cooked. It is low in starch and Diabetic friendly.

Cabbage

This is low in starch and Diabetic friendly. It does not contain any sugar.

Carrots

This must be eaten with the skin and also leaves, if you can source these. It is a non-starchy vegetable that is Diabetic friendly.

Organic Celery

This is very high in fibre and water content, has very low glycemic index, which can keep blood sugar in check.

Citrus fruits

Grapefruits, oranges, lemons, and limes are high in Vitamin C, folate and potassium which are important for overall Wellness.

Cucumber

This must be eaten with the skin. It is a non-starchy vegetable where you can satisfy your appetite.

Dandelion

This contains bioactive compounds that improve the secretion of insulin, the hormone that regulates blood sugar levels, as well as the absorption of glucose (sugar) in your muscles.

Fish

Fatty fish such as salmon, sardines, herring, mackerel, trout and tuna are high in Omega-3 and recommended for Diabetics. Choose grilled or baked instead of breaded and fried.

Kale

Dark leafy vegetables such as kale are packed with Vitamins A,C,E and K, iron, calcium, and potassium and beneficial for overall Wellness.

Nuts & Seeds

An ounce of nuts can go a long way in getting key healthy fats along with helping to manage hunger. Nuts are also high in magnesium and fibre. Walnuts and flaxseeds are high in Omega-3 fatty acids.

Please note that peanuts are NOT a nut. It is a legume and the most common allergy-causing foods and must be avoided. It is also a crop that is most heavily routinely saturated with pesticides.

Sea salt

This is recommended in place of the highly processed table salt.

Spinach

This is a non-starchy veggie, which means it does not have much effect on blood sugar levels. Young spinach leaves can be eaten raw and added to salads and sandwiches. It may also be cooked for few minutes on low heat or added to cooked foods when serving.

Sweet Potato

Although it tastes sweet, it has a sterling nutritional profile, making them a great food for Diabetics.

Whole grains

Such as oats, brown rice, red rice and wild rice are Diabetic friendly.

## *Contact Us*

If you or someone you know would like to have a discovery call with us, please book online via https://calendly.com/wellnessiridology

Or email us on hello@planetwellness.co.uk

Download our free guide Best Ways to Treat Diabetes:

https://planetwellness.co.uk/diabetesguide

You can connect with us on Facebook here:

Do also leave a review for us on Amazon so that others will be encouraged to read this book and learn from it.

Printed in Great Britain
by Amazon

24250623R00190